D1137903

Acupuncture: Techniques
Point Selection

Come, Memmius, lend a free ear and a shrewd mind, untrammelled by life's cares, to the study of the true doctrine; do not scorn the gifts prepared by my faithful friendship until you understand their worth, for it is a system encompassing both heaven and the gods that I intend to expose to you, and the principles of things that I am going to reveal to you . . .

Titus Lucretius
De Natura Rerum, Book One, 60 BC

Senior commissioning editor: Mary Seager
Development editor: Caroline Savage
Production controller: Anthony Read
Desk editor: Claire Hutchins
Cover designer: Helen Brockway

Acupuncture: Techniques for Successful Point Selection

Royston Low PhD DrAc ND DO MGOsC FBAcC

JET LIBRARY

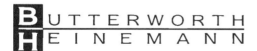

BUTTERWORTH
HEINEMANN

OXFORD AUCKLAND BOSTON JOHANNESBURG MELBOURNE NEW DELHI

Butterworth-Heinemann
Linacre House, Jordan Hill, Oxford OX2 8DP
225 Wildwood Avenue, Woburn, MA 01801-2041
A division of Reed Educational and Professional Publishing Ltd

A member of the Reed Elsevier plc group

First published 2001

© Reed Educational and Professional Publishing Ltd 2001

British Library Cataloguing in Publication Data
A catalogue record for this book is available from the British Library

Library of Congress Cataloguing in Publication Data
A catalogue record for this book is available from the Library of Congress

ISBN 0 7506 4852 X

Composition by Genesis Typesetting, Laser Quay, Rochester, Kent
Printed and bound by MPG Books Ltd, Bodmin, Cornwall

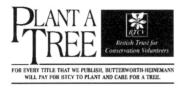

Contents

Introduction

In the past few years numerous books on acupuncture have poured out of China and from various other sources yet, with a few exceptions, nearly all have been 'the mixture as before', and nearly all have been based upon what is fondly called 'Traditional Chinese Medicine' (TCM). Yet very few question if this is the sum total of acupuncture, and not a single one gives an overall view of the actions of the points which might assist in the formulation of a treatment.

I can hear voices of dissent being raised from the protagonists of TCM – surely nearly all of the books give the reasons for the points selected: this one is good for internal wind, that one is good for stagnant blood, that for stimulating the lungs. To explain my heretical statements it is necessary to venture just a little into Chinese history to see how this has influenced the growth of acupuncture in the present day. Each of the various dynasties saw the development of particular fashions and approaches to medicine, each of the various philosophical schools changed and modified what had gone before and introduced new concepts, but the most important change of all was the recent one at the time of the so-called 'Dragon Empress', Tz'u-hsi (1835–1908). Her reign, beginning in 1861, saw the introduction of Western medicine into China and also brought about the fall of the Ching (Manchu) dynasty. This led to the establishment of the Republic of China (Guo Ming Dang) under Sun Yat Sen in 1911, and the virtual banning of acupuncture and traditional medicine in favour of the Western approach. The vastness of the country, coupled with the limited number of Western-trained doctors did, however, render this ultimately unfeasible, with the traditional medicine lingering on in the thousands of villages spread throughout the land. It also led to the migration of many of the leading practitioners of traditional medicine to Korea and Vietnam, to supplement the Chinese medicine which had already been taken to these countries (and to Japan) during the Tang period (618–907 AD).

With the inauguration of the People's Republic in 1949, and particularly with the beginning of that outstanding achievement, the Long March, the Republican Army found itself with an acute shortage of medicine and drugs, and immediate steps had to be taken to remedy this. Acupuncture and traditional medicine provided a ready answer, leading to Chairman Mao's famous dictum about Chinese medicine being a storehouse of knowledge, and that what was good was to be fostered and nourished and what was wrong or ineffective was to be discarded. Traditional medicine varied from Western medicine fundamentally in that its original approach was from a religio-philosophical viewpoint, and many of these earlier ideas were no longer tenable in a modern world, even if the techniques to which they gave rise were based upon decades of meticulous observation and were extremely workable. A quick and simple approach had to be devised – hence the conception of the 'bare-foot doctor' and the development of the 'Eight Approaches' system. Based on the underlying acceptance of the Yin/Yang concept and of the balance of opposites, this added the further dualities of Internal/External, Hot and Cold, and Excess and Deficiency, with every disease being considered as a permutation of combinations of these factors and symptoms brought about by internal or external pathogenic agents, the so-called Internal or External Devils. The practitioner arrived at a diagnosis based upon a differentiation of these symptoms to give a picture of a specific syndrome, to be treated by the use of specific points, herbs, and advice regarding lifestyle and diet as appropriate. This is the approach which today is known as Traditional Chinese Medicine, taught currently in schools in China and elsewhere under the misapprehension that this is the true and only form of 'traditional' acupuncture. The trouble is that it is based mainly upon a herbal concept and tries to equate the actions of specific points in a manner similar to the actions of specific herbs, i.e. this herb (or point) is good for internal heat, this herb (or point) will help to get the blood moving, etc., and whilst it is extremely helpful, even essential, for the treatment of the Zang/Fu (organs and viscera) and internal conditions, it is vastly inferior to other approaches when it comes to the treatment of musculo-skeletal and local conditions which are so prevalent in our Western practices.

TCM does of course make use of the Five Elements, or Five Phases, in its description of the relationship between the various organs and the vagaries of climate, emotion, etc. which affect them, and it acknowledges the actions of the Sheng (generative), Ko (controlling) and Wu (insulting) cycles, yet it teaches little of the manner of transference of energy on these cycles. Agreed, this concept was developed and fostered mainly by the Japanese, yet it is still a part of the true traditional teachings.

There is, however, one aspect of acupuncture which appears to be completely overlooked in TCM and which, in my opinion, is the most fundamental of all, the approach on which the whole of acupuncture is, or should be, based, namely the movement of energy.

To me, it is a matter for some amusement to consider that the Chinese antedated Einstein by some 2000 years with their original concept that matter and energy were interchangeable, and that matter was simply condensed energy. Following from this the human body is in itself basically energic in nature, 'dis-ease' is an imbalance in that energy and, in fact, all disease is caused by a 'stuckness', a lack of movement in that energy flow on one or more levels. As the quota of energy available in any one body at any one time is a constant, this implies that if the energy is not moving properly there will be an excess of energy built up on one side of the blockage and an accompanying deficit on the other – whether we are dealing with a Yin or Yang condition will depend upon the type of energy concerned. The aim of the practitioner is to establish where the blockage is, remove it, and get the energy flowing smoothly once more, to which end there are several different techniques and approaches available.

It is this aspect, dealing with an energic blockage, that seems to be missing from the present-day Chinese teaching, yet surely this is the basis of all true acupuncture, and it is this which has to a large extent survived in the Korean and Vietnamese teachings. Vietnamese practitioners have taken the knowledge to France, and it is inherent in the teachings of Chamfrault and Van Nghi. Allied to this attitude is a far more elaborate understanding of the movement of energy in the various channels. Although TCM pays lip service to the existence of the 'colaterals' and secondary vessels, their existence is hardly taken into account when it comes to treatment; even the Eight Extra meridians are used very little and certainly not to the extent that their great and deep action warrants.

A perfect understanding of how to use an acupuncture point will come only when we fully understand what a point is and how it acts, and this is still a long way beyond our present knowledge. The reader is referred to other books – mainly those by Pomeranz and Bensoussan – for a scientific discussion of the possible modus operandi of acupuncture points. Suffice it to say that their action is slowly being proven by Western medicine, and it is most likely by transmission via the hypothalamus with the consequential production of the various enkephalins, alpha and beta endorphins, serotonin, etc., and the stimulation of production of ACTH and other hormones. The fact that acupuncture can also stimulate the autoimmune system postulates a further effect upon the thymus gland. It is for these reasons that a sound knowledge of Western medicine as well as all aspects of Chinese medicine is essential for a properly qualified practitioner, who has to keep both aspects in mind when formulating his treatment plan.

Practically speaking, although we may not fully understand *how* the point works, this detail is not really important – after all, aspirin has been a medical standby for centuries, yet it is only very recently that we have discovered that its action is apparently by prostaglandin inhibition.

What we have to do is to assume that the original Chinese statements are true and act accordingly, whether we believe them or not, and we will find (often to our Western amazement) that it actually works.

The following chapters will detail the various approaches which have been followed.

The Five Elements (Five Phases)

Basic to the philosophy behind all Chinese medicine is the concept of the Five Elements, and the endeavour of the ancients to fit the properties of everything in nature into one of the five classifications.

The theory owed most of its inception to the so-called School of Naturalists (Yin-Yang Chia), its best known protagonist being Tsou Yen who lived (approximately) from 350 BC to 270 BC. According to Needham (1962, vol. 2, p. 238) it originally had reference to the ruling dynasties, each of which came under the jurisdiction of a particular element and the emperors of which actually clothed themselves in the colour appropriate to that element. (The Shen and Ko cycles – see later – made it difficult for any dynasty to believe that they could establish themselves in perpetuity, for the fluctuations in the cycle of the elements made any specific prognostication impossible.)

Needham's dissertation on the Five Elements (Needham, 1962, p. 244) is extremely interesting and is not mentioned in any of the standard Traditional Chinese Medicine (TCM) texts. He postulates their origin as suggesting the chemical interests of the Naturalists: the relationship of saltiness with Water was due to their observations on salination; and the bitterness of Fire arose from the use of heat in preparing herbal decoctions to produce bitter-tasting substances, and also the combination of hot and bitter tastes in spices. The association of sourness with Wood came from the observation that as vegetation decomposed it produced a sour odour – the alkali in plant ashes was also sour tasting. Acridity in Metal arose from the acrid fumes produced during smelting operations, whilst sweetness was associated with Earth because of the sweet taste of many cereals and also, possibly, from the finding of bees' nests, containing honey, in the earth.

Of course if this were true, the effect of the various flavoured foods upon the organs subtended by the corresponding elements, i.e. sourness affecting the liver, sweet affecting the spleen, would be basically imaginary. The fact that salt can affect fluid retention is possibly purely fortuitous!

Even the well-known cycle of energy was subject to much speculation in the early days – Needham states that there was a total of 36 possible variations postulated by various writers, but four major ones:

The Cosmogenic (Seng hsü)	Wa	F	Wo	M	E
The Mutual Production (Hsiang sêng)	Wo	F	E	M	Wa
The Mutual Conquest (Hsiang shêng)	Wo	M	F	Wa	
The Modern	M	Wo	Wa	F	E

The Cosmogenic is the evolutionary order in which the elements were supposed to come into being; the Mutual Production the order in which the Five Elements were supposed to produce each other; and the Mutual Conquest the series in which each element was supposed to conquer its predecessor (this is possibly the oldest of all, as it is the one associated with Tsou Yen himself). No explanation is given for the Modern order, but it occurs in such important texts as Kuo Yü, Pai Hu Thung Tê Lun, etc.

The Mutual Production is, of course, the well-known Sheng cycle, but the Mutual Conquest is the reverse Ko or Wu cycle. From extensions of this one arrives at the two principles, of control (Hsiang chi) and masking (Hsiang hua).

Control (Ko cycle):
 1 Wood destroys (conquers) Earth, but Metal controls the process.
 4 Metal destroys (conquers) Wood, but Fire controls the process.
 2 Fire destroys (conquers) Metal, but Water controls the process.
 5 Water destroys (conquers) Fire, but Earth controls the process.
 3 Earth destroys (conquers) Water, but Wood controls the process.

(Metal destroys Wood by cutting it up, but Fire controls by melting the Metal faster than it can cut up the Wood.)

Masking:
 Wood destroys Earth, but Fire masks the process.
 Fire destroys Metal, but Earth masks the process.
 Earth destroys Water, but Metal masks the process.
 Metal destroys Wood, but Water masks the process.
 Water destroys Fire, but Wood masks the process.

(Water 'masks' by producing Wood faster than the Metal can cut it up.)

The origin of the medical correlations is obscure. They are given in the Nei Ching, and it appears that the bulk of the text is from the early Han, and some possibly from the Warring States period, but it may be assumed that the theory of the Five Phases, the Wu Xing, is essentially part of the Taoist philosophy and is part of the concept, essential to

Chinese thought, that Man is a replica of the Universe (mirroring the Hermetic 'as above, so below') and that the flow of Qi through his body corresponds to the movements of the force of life in large segments of nature.

Originally there were four basic elements based on the four points of the compass. In Chinese maps the cartographer always stood facing the sun, i.e. the South, so that the South was always at the top of the map, with the East on his left and the West on his right, with the North behind him, whilst he himself was on the Earth in the centre (making the fifth element) (Fig. 1.1).

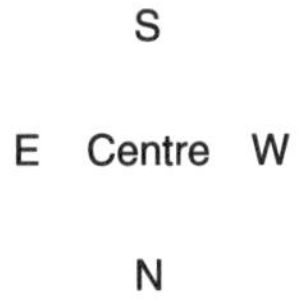

S

E   Centre   W

N

Figure 1.1

As the sun rises in the East to open and enliven the day, so the yearly energy begins in the East, which is therefore given the designation of Spring. The energy increases to a maximum in Summer and then slowly declines through Autumn, goes deep, and encapsulates itself in the Winter, to regenerate itself in the next Springtime. We can thus add to the diagram shown in Fig. 1.1 to get Fig. 1.2.

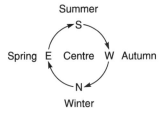

Figure 1.2

- The Spring and the East stand for birth and growth – element Wood.
- The Summer and the South stand for climax and maturity – element Fire.
- The Autumn and the West stand for balance and harvest – element Earth.
- The Winter and the North stand for emptiness and storage – element Water.

As we have seen, the fifth element is the Earth upon which Man is based, and an old book, the Hong Fan, describes the energy circuit as shown in Fig. 1.3.

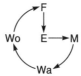

Figure 1.3

This soon transformed into the cycle shown in Fig. 1.4, which is the formation familiar to all acupuncturists and is the Mutual Production cycle mentioned earlier.

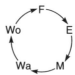

Figure 1.4

Seasonally, because it takes up a position between Summer and Autumn, Earth is regarded as Long Summer, otherwise known in North America as Fall.

Although the actual origin of the medical correlations is unclear, the Chinese theory of the Universe declared that the Five Elements were the basis of all matter, and the Chinese mind, unfettered by Aristotelian logic, reasoned that the human body necessarily was no exception. For the Chinese, the function was more important than the organ which produced it – the organ was the shadowy 'power behind the throne', but it was through the function that the organ manifested itself and had its reason for being.

Of the organs, five were the originators of all movement within the body – the liver, heart, spleen, lungs and kidneys. They were solid and, like Winter, they stored the energy. Their characteristics were Yin, and they were known as the Zang. These Zang organs had to have their Yang (Fu) counterpart, which unlike the Yin organs periodically filled and emptied and eliminated substances, and these were respectively the Gall Bladder, Small Intestines, Stomach, Colon and Bladder.

The Chinese regarded the liver as the first organ. Armed only with intuition and perception they realized its function of regulating the flow of blood and nourishment in the body, and equated this with the stirring of life in the wood of Springtime. The redness and warmth of the blood it pumped naturally put the heart under the rulership of Fire; the nourishment provided by stomach and spleen was as central to Man's existence as the earth on which he was founded. The spleen generates the lungs, which correspond to the element Metal, sometimes translated as Air. The fifth of the Zang organs is the kidneys. They are black, taste salty and have a putrid odour. The Chinese concept of kidneys also covers the adrenal glands, with which they are in close anatomical relationship, and this accounts for the kidneys 'ruling the bones' and for their general extreme importance.

According to Chinese medical theory there are two further organs, or rather functions, within the body. They are the Pericardium, which is the Zang aspect, and the Three Heaters, which is the Fu. They come under the rulership of Fire, the Heart and Small Intestine being regarded as Fire Prince, and the Pericardium and Triple Heaters as the Fire Minister. The major correspondences are given in Table 1.1.

Table 1.1 Five Element Correspondences

	Element				
	Wood	*Fire*	*Earth*	*Metal*	*Water*
Direction	East	South	Centre	West	North
Colour	Green	Red	Yellow	White	Black
Season	Spring	Summer	Long summer	Autumn	Winter
Climate	Wind	Heat	Humidity	Dryness	Cold
Process	Birth	Growth	Maturity	Harvest	Storage
Nourishes	Muscles	Blood vessels	Flesh	Skin	Bones
Expands into	Nails	Colour	Lips	Body hair	Head hair
Orifice	Eyes	Tongue	Mouth	Nose	Ears
Sense	Sight	Speech	Taste	Smell	Hearing
Flavour	Sour	Bitter	Sweet	Pungent	Salt
Body smell	Rancid	Scorched	Fragrant	Rank	Putrid
Liquid	Tears	Sweat	Saliva	Mucus	Urine
Emotion	Aggression	Joy	Calmness	Sympathy	Caution
Excess emotion	Anger	Over-excitement	Depression	Grief	Fear
Human sound	Shout	Laughter	Singing	Weeping	Groaning
Chinese note	Chio	Chih	Kung	Shang	Yu
Meat	Chicken	Mutton	Beef	Horse	Pork
Cereal	Wheat	Rice	Maize	Oats	Beans

Sheng cycle transference

We have seen that there is a natural cycle of regeneration inherent in this concept of 5-Element energy balances, and this is known as the Sheng cycle or Mother–Son relationship. In this instance Wood is the mother of Fire, which in turn is the son of Wood and the mother of Earth. Earth is the mother of Metal, which is the son of Earth and the mother of Water, and so on. It is to be noted that the energy flows in one direction – clockwise – *only*. (For the moment we will concern ourselves only with the Zang or Yin organs, as these are the important ones. Effects on the Fu, or hollow organs are usually purely secondary.)

Four pathological states can arise from this:

1 Hyperfunction (Shi) of the mother can cause an excess of energy to be transferred to the son.
2 Hypofunction (Xu) in the mother can result in a deficiency of energy in the son.
3 Hypofunction in the son can draw excessively upon the mother and will cause a deficiency in that organ, or
4 Hyperfunction in the son can cause a 'back pressure' or blockage on the Sheng cycle, thus preventing the normal flow of energy out of the mother and again causing disease in that organ.

To correct an imbalance we always try to transfer from where there is an excess of energy to a deficiency, which means that if the son is weak we will endeavour to 'pull' energy from the mother. We do this by stimulating the so-called 'tonification point' of the deficient meridian, this point being the point pertaining to the element which is the mother of the organ being dealt with, i.e. to pull energy from Fire to Earth we tonify the Fire point of the Earth meridian (Sp2), and the Earth point of Metal (Lu9) to pull from Earth to Metal (Fig. 1.5).

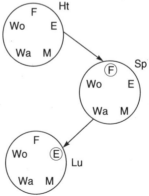

Figure 1.5

Note that there is no drainage or dispersal on Sheng cycle transference, and that energy is always taken from an excess to fill a deficit. This being the case, one cannot draw from an 'excess' organ into a normal one – one can only work to fill a deficiency. Therefore,

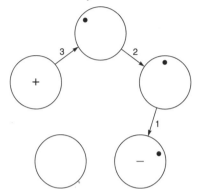

Figure 1.6

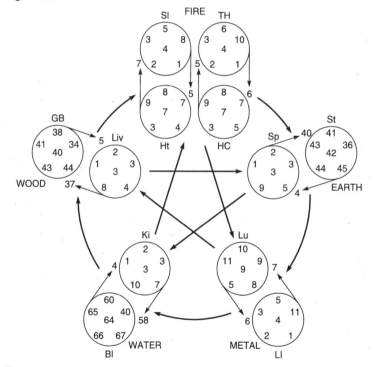

Figure 1.7

to draw from Wood to Metal one has to work backwards, starting by filling the deficiency in Metal by toning the Earth point of Metal (Fig. 1.6 and Fig. 1.7 on page 7).

This creates a temporary deficiency in Earth, which is filled by stimulating the Fire point of Earth, now creating a temporary deficiency in Fire. This is replenished by stimulating the Wood point of Fire, which drains the aberrant excess out of Wood. Note that *one cannot work backwards* on the Sheng cycle, i.e. go against the natural energy flow and pull from Wood to Water, etc.

So far we have dealt only with disorders with the Zang organs. Imbalances can also arise in the Fu. If the imbalance is purely within the Yang orbit, for example between Gall Bladder and Stomach, one proceeds as above but uses the Yang meridians. That is, if GB+, St−, one stimulates the Fire point of Stomach and then the Wood point of Small Intestine.

But it is possible for an imbalance to occur within a Yin and a Yang couple, for example between Gall Bladder and Liver or Lungs and Colon, and here we make the acquaintance of two other points – the Luo point and the Yuan or Source point. To maintain the energy balance in each pair of coupled meridians there is the Transverse Luo vessel, which runs from the Luo point of one meridian to the Yuan point of the other, and here things become a little more complicated (Fig. 1.8).

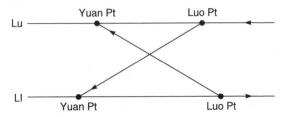

Figure 1.8

Shortly we will see that we have to decide between relative degrees of aberrance, but for the moment we will abide by the simple rule of always 'pulling' from an excess, and in this instance the rule is 'Take the appropriate action upon the Yuan point of the aberrant meridian and the opposite action upon the Luo point of the coupled meridian', i.e. in the case of Lu+ we would sedate the Yuan point of Lu and tonify the Luo point of LI. In the case of LI− we would sedate the Luo point of Lu and tonify the Yuan point of LI (Fig. 1.9).

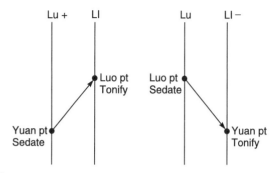

Figure 1.9

Consider the Sheng cycle imbalance depicted in Fig. 1.10 as an example.

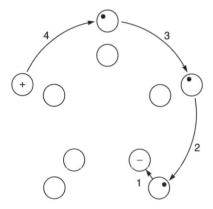

Figure 1.10

As we must always work to fill a deficit, our primary target would be to supply the empty Lu. We have Lu− and LI normal, therefore we take the appropriate action upon the Yuan point of Lu and tonify it, whilst draining the Luo point of LI. We have thus created a temporary deficit in Colon, which we fill by the normal Mother–Son technique as seen previously – to Earth point of LI, Fire point of St, Wood point of SI.

Another example is shown in Fig. 1.11.

Here one would tonify the Yuan point of Bl, sedate the Luo point of Ki, and tonify the Metal point of Ki and the Earth point of Lu.

It is, of course, theoretically possible to cross the Yin/Yang barrier at any other place, as shown in Fig. 1.12. Here one would tonify the Metal

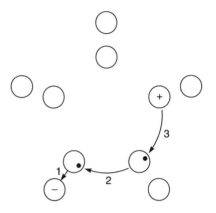

Figure 1.11

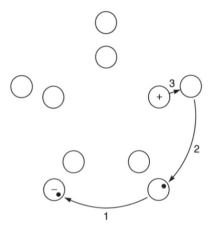

Figure 1.12

point of Bl, Earth point of LI, then sedate the Yuan point of Sp and tonify the Luo point of St.

However, as I have stated in my book on the Secondary Vessels (Low, 1983), the most important thing to remember in the use of the Transverse Luo vessels is that they are concerned with the regulation of the internal Jung energy balance and *not* with perverse energy. If one meridian should be in a state of fullness because of the presence of perverse energy, then the worst thing one could possibly do would be to transfer that perverse energy into the unaffected meridian. As this discrimination is so important, a few of the major differentiations are listed in Table 1.2.

Table 1.2 Symptoms related to perverse energy and internal causes

	Perverse energy	Internal causes
Lu	Dyspnoea Fullness of lungs Pains in apex of lungs	Fullness in chest Sensation of uprising energy Cough Asthma Palms of hands hot
LI	Swollen neck Ache in teeth	Dryness of mouth and throat Pain along pathway When very empty – shivering
St	Darkish complexion Photophobia Wants to be left alone Borborygmus	Fever with sweating Catarrh Oedema of throat Abdominal distension Pains along pathway When over-full – heat in stomach and chest, over-quick digestion, dark urine When very empty – cold in stomach and chest, stomach swollen
Sp	Abdominal distension with belching, better after passing flatus Vomiting immediately after meals Stiffness at root of tongue	Diarrhoea Pain in cardiac area Body feels stiff Pain at root of tongue Disturbance on pathway
Ht	Dry throat with thirst Cardiac pain, worse 11.00 p.m. – 1.00 a.m.	Pains on pathway Eyes yellowish
SI	Acute pains on pathway	Pain in whole pathway Tinnitus and/or deafness Submaxillary swelling
Bl	Pains on pathway Bulging eyes Sensation of rising energy Headaches	Sharp pains along pathway Sharp pains in head and neck Eyes yellowish Lacrimation Haemorrhoids
Ki	Dark complexion Cough, dyspnoea Very hungry, but cannot eat Visual disturbances Fearful and anxious	Pains along pathway Legs cold and numb Sensation of rising energy Throat and tongue dry, mouth hot Diarrhoea Grief, desire to lie down

Table 1.2 continued

	Perverse energy	Internal causes
Pe	Palm of hand hot, with pain on pathway Ruddy complexion False laughter	Palm of hand hot Circulatory disturbances Pain in heart Grief
TH	Sore throat Tinnitus and/or deafness	Pain on pathway Perspiration
GB	Bitter taste in mouth Outside of leg hot, chest and side painful Frequent sighing	Pains on pathway, particularly affecting the joints Sweating and shivering
Liv	Pain in kidney area with stiffness in spine Genital affections Possible dry throat	Indigestion with nausea and vomiting Fullness in chest Diarrhoea Either weak bladder or difficulty in passing urine

The Four Needle Technique

This is an extremely useful technique which is called for *only* when there is an imbalance on the Ko cycle, for example Liv+, Sp−, when Spleen is deficient *because* Liver is overactive and is exerting too much control over it. It is therefore logical to sedate Liver in order to decrease this control and allow Spleen to increase. The rule is to work first on the 'opposition' or *controlling* organ on the Ko cycle, and we first take the appropriate action on the *element point of the element* (i.e. the Water point of Ki, Metal point of Lu, etc.) using the element point of the controlling organ on both control and subject. In the example given, our first step is to sedate the Wood point of Liver (Liv1) and also the Wood point of Spleen (Sp1). But our subject, the Spleen, is underactive, so we follow up with the second part of the treatment by stimulating the mother of the spleen, which is Heart, on its element point (the Fire point, Ht8) and also the Fire point of Spleen (Sp2).

If, on the other hand, the Liver had been underactive and allowed the Spleen to develop too much energy, then we would have had to stimulate the Liver and we would thus tonify Liv1 and Sp1. However, this time we need to sedate the Spleen, and we do this by draining or reducing the son – the Lungs – again on their own element points, so we sedate the Metal point of Lungs, Lu8, and the Metal point of Spleen, Sp5.

Table 1.3 shows specimen treatments for the first four meridians – it is suggested that the reader works out the remainder of the meridians for him or herself to get the hang of it.

Table 1.3

Meridian	Full		Empty	
	1 Tonify	2 Sedate	1 Sedate	2 Tonify
Lu	Lu10,Ht8	Ki10, Lu5	Lu10 Ht8	Lu9, Sp3
LI	LI5, SI5	Bl66, LI2	LI5, SI5	LI11, St36
St	St43, GB41	LII, St45	St43, GB41	SI5, St41
Sp	Liv1, Sp1	Lu8, Sp5	Liv1, Sp1	Ht8, Sp2

All points are used bilaterally. It must be stressed that this technique is used *only* when it is specifically called for on the Ko cycle. On no account must any excess be 'pulled' across the Ko cycle, i.e. Liv+, Sp–, stimulate Sp1, as this would serve only to exacerbate the condition.

2
The 'Welling' Theory

Parallel with the consideration of the transfer of energy on the Five-Element cycle is an understanding of the way in which the energy flows in the meridians. The flow of energy in the 24-hour cycle is familiar to all practitioners (Fig. 2.1).

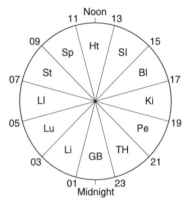

Figure 2.1

Figure 2.2 not only illustrates the union of the paired Yin and paired Yang meridians to make up the six jiaos, but also shows the Yin/Yang couples – Lu/LI, St/Sp, etc.

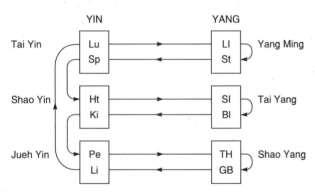

Figure 2.2

All the so-called 'antique' or 'command' points are towards the distal ends of the meridians, where the energy is at its most mutable, i.e. Yin is becoming more Yang and vice versa, and is in the superficial zone before going deep at the Ho point. The Welling Theory is so called because, traditionally, the energy is supposed to 'bubble up' like water from a well, at the Tsing point (will the reader please note that in this one particular instance I prefer the use of the Wade–Giles transliteration of Tsing, Yong, Yu, Ching, Ho rather than the Pinyin Jing, Ying, Shu, Jing, He, simply because differentiation is easier!), gradually becoming stronger as it flows towards the depths of the body, just as a river, starting as a trickle, gathers strength and volume on its journey to the sea. The five points can be briefly explained as follows:

1 **Tsing point (the Well)**. This is the point where the basic energy flow is at its weakest, in that the Yin/Yang balance between the coupled meridians is at its most mutable. Depending upon the particular meridian, it is either the point of departure of the energy or of its arrival. It is also the point where the Wei energy is taken in from the Tendino-Muscular meridian and from where the Wei energy in its turn is strengthened from the main meridian.

2 **Yong point (the Spring)**. Traditionally regarded as the 'increased force of flow' because the energy from the coupled meridian tends to react more strongly at this point, with Yin becoming Yang or Yang becoming Yin.

3 **Yu point (the Stream)**. The flow becomes stronger. Traditionally, the point 'transports' and 'directs' the energy, whilst the perverse energy is absorbed into the general meridial stream for transportation elsewhere.

4 **Yuan point (River Junction)**. The energy of the Transverse Luo vessels flows in at this point thereby strengthening the general flow if required and giving energy to turn the 'Stream' into a 'River'. It is said to absorb the Wei defensive energy, but as in reality the Wei energy is simply the defensive aspect of the basic body potential, the correct meaning is that the defensive capabilities are enhanced by the increased potential available. (Note that in a Yin meridian the functions of the Yu and Yuan points are combined in the Yu point.)

5 **Ching point (the River)**. Known as the point 'of crossing and deviation', this is the point where the energy concentrates and from where the perverse energy may be 'disembarked for storage elsewhere', i.e. a 'perverse influence' (e.g. an inflammatory reaction) if it reaches this point can spread into the neighbouring bones, muscles or joints or can even affect a neighbouring meridian.

6 **Ho point (the Sea)**. The point where the energy goes from the superficial to the deeper levels or vice versa, therefore known as the

point of entry or exit. In the distal portion of the meridian the energy is, as we have seen, in a state of flux. Proximal to the Ho point it becomes deeper and more of a definite Yin or Yang, although as even these terms are descriptive of action it may be preferable to think of it as Yong energy, the deep potential of the meridian.

(It is of interest to note that according to the oldest traditions the Heart meridian has no Yu point. This is because the Yu point is the point of absorption of perverse energy, and if perverse energy reached the heart it would mean inevitable death. Accordingly, the perverse energy reaches only the Pericardium or Fire Minister and cannot enter the Fire Prince.)

As the energy from the coupled meridian flows in at the Tsing point, it reaches a maximum at the Yong point, then partakes more of its particular Yin or Yang characteristics until flowing deep into the 'Sea' at the Ho point (Fig. 2.3).

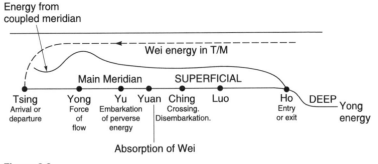

Figure 2.3

It is interesting to note that its entry into a Yin meridian is more gradual, as in Fig. 2.4, whilst in a Yang meridian the energy tends to build up at the Ho point before going deep, as in Fig. 2.5, which is why the Ho point of a Yang meridian has a stronger action than that of a Yin meridian.

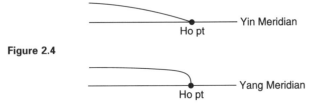

Figure 2.4

Figure 2.5

We have also noted that the inflowing energy reaches a peak at the Yong point – this coupled inflowing energy is Yang in a Yin meridian and vice versa. In a Yin meridian, which starts cyclically on Wood or Springtime, the Yong point corresponds to Summer, which is when the Yang energy peaks. In a Yang meridian (starting on Metal or Autumn) the Yong point corresponds to Winter, the time of maximum Yin.

When discussing the Five-Element character of the points, we have already dealt with the use of the five antique or Shu points for tonification or draining according to the promoting relationship of the Five Elements. However, of particular importance is their relationship to the pathogenic factors of Wind, Heat, Damp, Dryness and Cold (Table 2.1).

Table 2.1 The Actions of Command Points

Element	Point	Pathogenic factor	Actions
Wood	All Yin Wood points	Wind	To expel Internal Wind
Fire	Ht8 Lu10	Heat	Expels Summer Heat or Fire in Heart Expels Wind-Heat or Empty-Fire from Yin Xu condition
	Pe8 Liv2 Sp2 Ki2	Fire	Expels Summer Heat or Fire Subdues Liver Fire NOT to reduce Heat (Sp has no Fire) To reduce Empty Fire from Ki Yin Xu and to cool blood
Earth	Ht7 Pe7 Lu9 Sp3 Liv3 Ki3	Dampness/ Phlegm	NOT to expel phlegm To expel phlegm from Heart Expels phlegm from Lungs To resolve Dampness To resolve Dampness or Phlegm NOT to resolve Dampness (no syndrome of Damp in Kidney)
Water	Ht3 Pe3 Lu5 Liv8 Sp9 Ki10	Cold	Not to expel Cold To reduce Heat in Blood Expels Cold and Heat from Lungs (Internal) Expels Damp-Cold from Lower Heater Expels Damp-Cold and Damp-Heat from Lower Heater Expels Damp-Cold from Lower Heater

Note: No Metal or Dryness, as Dryness is an imbalance on Water.

This is important for two reasons:

- the powerful action of the five Shu points on the channel and the organ as compared to that of the points on the head and trunk;
- they can treat diseases of the Zang/Fu (as distal points), whilst points on the head, chest and trunk treat mainly local areas.

As we have seen, according to the Welling Theory each channel is seen as a river, with different levels of progression from deep to superficial, from far to near, and from small to big. This progression has nothing to do with the direction of the channel.

According to the Nan Ching (the third part of the *Nei Ching*) in Chapter 68, each Shu point shares a common action irrespective of channel or element.

1	Tsing	For fullness under the heart, mental restlessness.
2	Yong	Heat in the body, heat diseases; all expel heat.
3	Yu	Feeling of heaviness, joints ache, Bi syndrome due to damp.
4	Ching	Panting, cough, throat, asthma, intermittent fever, hot and cold sensations.
5	Ho	Rebellious Qi and diarrhoea; treats the Fu organs, gastric and intestinal problems.

Use of the Shu (antique) points according to the Nan Ching

Tsing

- Applies to both Yin and Yang channels.
- Strong action on the brain.
- 'Usually reducing action, bringing Fire down'.
- Emergencies like Windstroke, to restore consciousness.
- Mental restlessness caused by Fire in the top (Ki1, Sp1, Ht9).

Yong

- Nearly all points to expel Heat.
- Applies to both Yin and Yang channels, but particularly to Yin.
- Stronger effect than the Tsing points.
- Yin channels – all are reducing points (Foot Yong points stronger than Hand Yong points).

● 'Energy gushes through from Tsing (Well) point' – very dynamic points.

Liv2 to expel Liver Fire.
Ki2 to expel Empty Fire from Kidney.
Lu10 Lung phlegm heat, hot dry throat.
Pe8 and Ht8: when Heart Fire to be subdued.
Yang channels: St44 to subdue Stomach Heat; GB43 to subdue Gall Bladder Heat.

Yu

● Applies to both Yin and Yang channels, particularly to Yang.
● For Bi syndrome, dampness.
● LI3, SI3 and TH3 for Bi syndrome affecting the hands.
● St43 for generalized Bi syndrome of body.

Sp3

● *The* point to reduce and resolve dampness.

Ching

● Applies to both Yin and Yang channels, particularly to the Yin.
● Applies to some points particularly on the Yang channel of the Yang Ming.
● LI5 and St41 to reduce Fire from Yang Ming affecting the throat.

Ho

● Applies to both Yin and Yang channels, but especially the Yang, and particularly the lower Ho points for the Fu.

St37: Lower Ho for colon (can be used to tonify the according Fu).
St39: Lower Ho for Small Intestine (can be used to tonify the according Fu).
Bl39: Lower Ho for Lower Heater (can be used to tonify the according Fu).
Bl40: GB34, St36: can be used together to tonify the Fu organs.
St37: expels Damp-Heat from intestines; chronic diarrhoea; chronic intestinal problems.
St39: lower abdominal pain.
Bl39: important point for treating the Lower Heater; oedema of leg; expels Cold-Damp or Damp-Heat; regulates urination – too much (Ki Yang Xu), tonify; too little (Shi condition), reduce.

- For the Yin channels:

  Sp9, Liv8, Ki10: diarrhoea from Damp-Heat or Cold-Damp – use points to disperse it.

  Pe3, LI11, TH10: regulate the intestines.

Ling Shu, (the second part of the *Nei Ching*, Chapter 4)

- Yong and Yu points – to treat disorders of the exterior.
- Ho points (especially lower) – to treat disorders of the interior, and Fu organs.

Ling Shu, (the second part of the *Nei Ching*, Chapter 6)

- Ho points – treat Yang in Yang, i.e. skin and muscles.
- Ching points – treat Yin in Yang, i.e. tendons and bones.
- Lower Ho points – treat Yang in Yin, i.e. Fu organs.
- Yong and Yu points (of Yin channels) – treat Yin in Yin, i.e. Zang organs.

Table 2.2 Summary

Points	Yin channels	Yang channels
Tsing	(a) Mental restlessness (b) When Zang organs affected (c) To expel internal wind	(a) Mental restlessness
Yong	(a) Heat diseases (b) Illnesses having a repercussion on the complexion (c) To treat Zang (with Yu point) (d) To expel Heat, Fire	(a) Heat diseases (b) To treat exterior disease (with the Yu point) (c) To expel heat
Yu	(a) For joint pains (b) Illnesses alternating between amelioration and aggravation (c) To treat the Zang (with Yong point) (d) To resolve Dampness	(a) For joint pains (b) Illnesses alternating as with the Yin (c) For exterior disease (with Yong point) (d) For Bi syndrome
Ching	(a) For cough, etc. (b) For illnesses affecting voice (c) Disease in tendons and bones	(a) For cough, etc. (b) For illnesses affecting voice (c) Disease in tendons and bones (d) To expel Heat
Ho	(a) To treat 'rebellious Qi' diarrhoea (b) To expel cold	(a) For disease of the exterior, skin, muscles

Clinical use of the other Shu points

Yuan ('Source') points

The 12 Yuan points are related to the Yuan Qi. Each of the Zang organs contains some Yuan Qi which theoretically shows at the Yuan point. If any of the five Zang are diseased, traditionally (but unfortunately seldom in practice!) abnormal reactions will appear at the corresponding Yuan points in the form of swelling, redness, congested blood vessels, varicose veins, deep sunken effect (around Ki3), bluish colour or flaccid skin tone.

The Yuan points should thus be usable for diagnosis to tell us which Zang organs are diseased, and treatment would include the use of the Yuan point.

Nan Ching (the third part of the *Nei Ching*, Chapter 66) states:

- The Yuan points are related to the Yuan Qi.
- The Yuan Qi originates between the two kidneys, at Ming Men. Yuan Qi passes through the three jiaos, spreads to the Zang/Fu and the 12 Jingluo. The places where the Yuan Qi stays are the Yuan points.
- Yuan point: most important point of the channel to tonify Yang; has an important action on Yuan Qi.
- New interpretation of the San Jiao: Avenue of Yuan Qi. Yuan Qi has an effect upon the body via the San Jiao.

Ling Shu (the second part of the *Nei Ching*, Chapter 1):

- Gives the Yuan points as Lu9, Pe7, Liv3, Ki3 (no Ht, as Ht and Pe were considered as one), but also CV15 was given as the Yuan point for Gao (fat) – it was stated that the Yuan Qi of fatty tissues gathers at CV15, whilst CV6 was given as the Yuan point for Huang (membranes) and the Yuan Qi for these gathers at CV6.
- The Yuan points are given as the main points to tonify the Zang (also the Back Shu points), whilst the Lower Ho points are given as the main points to tonify the Fu.

Luo points

There are two main considerations to bear in mind:

- Each Luo channel connects with an internal and an external channel.
- It departs from the Luo point along a specific pathway.

The Luo channel has two different uses:

1 In conjunction with the Yuan point of its coupled meridian, the energy from the Luo point will strengthen the energy in its coupled Yuan point. For example:
  For Lu, Lu9 Yuan point and LI6 as Luo point.
  For LI, LI4 Yuan point and Lu7 as Luo point.
2 On its own. For this we must know the pathway of the Luo channel and be able to distinguish whether it is in a Shi or a Xu condition and treat accordingly. (An obscure quotation in the Nan Ching states that when the Luo channels are full they can be seen, but not when they are empty, but see Low (1983) for a fuller analysis of both the Longitudinal and Transverse Luos.)

Du Mai Luo point: GV1

● Controls all the Yang Luo channels of the body.
● Shi: pain and stiffness in the spine.
● Xu: dizziness.

Ren Mai Luo point: CV15

● Controls all the Yin Luo channels of the body.
● Shi: pain on the skin of the abdomen.
● Xu: itching on the skin of the abdomen.

Great Luo of the Spleen: Sp21

● Controls all the blood of the body.
● Shi: pain all over the body.
● Xu: weakness in muscles and limbs *or* loosening of all the articulations with weakness and loss of strength in all joints.

The pathway of the Luo channel explains some of the actions of these points, as does its coupled action. For example:

Lu7: Action on the shoulder by virtue of the LI channel.
St40: Stomach problems, but also strengthens Sp and St. Resolves phlegm and damp.
Pe6: Special point for the chest.
TH5: Essential point for Wind/Heat, and to relieve exterior symptoms.

Xi – cleft points (accumulation points)

These are added points in acute problems. The meaning of Xi is a hole, fissure or crack, and it is the point on the channel where the blood and Qi meet. These points are used for acute painful inflammatory diseases of the Zang/Fu, especially the organs as opposed to the channels, and for situations where the blood and Qi are out of balance, especially the blood (haemoptysis, epistaxis).

In acute painful disease, where stagnation of blood causes severe pain, the Xi point will release the stagnation and thus relieve the pain. (The points Ht6 'Yinxi' and Pe4 'Ximen' include the word Xi because of their close relation with the heart and thus the blood.)

Lu6 Kong Zui (Opening Maximum)

● Regulates blood and bleeding.
● Eliminates heat.
● Characteristic symptoms: sore throat, loss of voice, haemoptysis, epistaxis, cough, shortness of breath.
● All full and hot Lu conditions: acute cough, stuffy chest.

LI7 Wen Liu (Warm Slide)

● Not much used.
● Cools heat, disperses excess in the tongue.

St34 Liang Qiu (Ridge Mound)

● Severe abdominal pain, acute stomach problems.
● Pain in the upper half of the abdomen, periumbilical pain.
● Harmonizes the stomach and nourishes the channel.
● Swelling and pain in the breasts, acute mastitis.

Sp8 Di Ji (Earth's Mechanism)

● An important point in menstrual problems.
● Acute pain – adjusts and harmonizes the Qi and blood, moves the blood.
● Adjusts the uterus, acute dysmenorrhoea, stabbing pain, pain due to clots in uterine blood.

Ht6 Yin Xi (Yin Xi)

● Acute pain, cools the Heart, absorbs Yin, sinks floating Yang, pacifies the Spirit.
● Important point in sweating.
● Epistaxis, haemoptysis, endometritis, night sweats, chest pain – all due to blood stagnation.
● Important for Yin Xu conditions, especially in hot flushes.

SI6 Yang Lao (Nourish the Old)

- Stiff neck.
- Moves the channel.
- Brightens the eyes.
- Relaxes the tendons.

Bl63 Jinmen (Golden Door)

- Secondary point.
- Torticollis, low back pain in the elderly.

Ki5 Shui Quan (Spring)

- Secondary point.
- Adjusts the menses, disperses congestion in the lower jiao, benefits the throat and eyes, amenorrhoea, uterine prolapse, retention of urine, premenstrual tension – all due to stagnation.

Pe4 Xi Men (Gate of the Crevice)

- Emergency point in acute heart attack; good for a lot of heart problems.
- Regulates Qi and Blood in the channel.
- Quietens the heart, pacifies the spirit, cools the blood, relaxes the chest.

TH7 Hui Zong (Meeting of the Clan)

- Sudden deafness (stagnation of Qi).

GB36 Wai Qiu (Outer Mound)

- Secondary point.
- Hepatitis, sciatica when tender.

Li6 Zhong Du (Middle Metropolis)

- Not much used.
- Adjusts Qi and Blood, stops pain in the lower abdomen.
- Symptoms of retained placenta and hernia (Li governs the lower abdomen).

Ki9 Zhu Bin (House Guest)

- Affects the spirit, nephritis, cystitis, orchitis.

GB35 Yang Jiao (Yang's Intersection)

● Mainly for acute lumbar sprain.

Ki8 Jiao Xin (Communicate Belief)

● Adjusts the menses.

Bl59 Fu Yang (Tarsal Yang)

● Benefits the eyes.

Back Shu points, Front Mu points

● Both treat the organs as opposed to the channels.
● Can be used in diagnosis by palpation.
● Back Shu points – more for tonifying the Zang organs because they suffer from weakness.
● Front Mu points – more for the Fu, which usually suffer from obstruction.
● Moxa is often used on both. For the Back Shu, often after the disease is cured, when we then reinforce with moxa.
● Needle the Back Shu points towards the spine.

The most common combinations are:

Bl18 and Liv14 – for liver problems, acute gallstones.
Bl23 and GB25 – kidney stones, kidney infection.
CV3 and Bl28 – for all bladder problems, urinary infection.

Back Shu points

Bl13 Fei Shu (Lu) (Lung's Hollow)

● All lung problems – full or empty, hot or cold.
● Adjusts and regulates Lu Qi.
● Clears Perverse Energy – Wind-Heat, Wind-Cold.
● Tonifies weakness.
● Clears both Full and Empty Heat.
● Stops cough.
● Not too deep insertion, especially with patient with weak lungs.

Bl14 Jue Yin Shu (Pe) (Absolute Yin Hollow)

● Not much used.

Bl15 Xin Shu (Ht) (Heart's Hollow)

- Frequently used.
- Nourishes the Heart, pacifies the Spirit, moves Ht Blood and Qi.
- Moves all Qi and Blood.
- Palpitations, shortness of breath, vomiting, madness.

Bl16 Du Shu (GV) (Governing Hollow)

- Not much used.
- Brings the Jing to the head – baldness!

Bl17 Ge She (Diaphragm's Hollow)

- Regulates Blood, transforms congealed blood.
- Expands chest and diaphragm.
- Strengthens deficiency conditions.

Bl18 Gan Shu (Liv) (Liver's Hollow)

- Comforts the Liver, benefits the Gall Bladder, disperses Heat (Li Yang rising) and Damp-Heat (hepatitis).
- Nourishes the Blood, clears the head, brightens the eyes.
- Quietens the Spirit, both dispersing excess (heat of Li) and tonifying the Blood.

Bl19 Dan Shu (GB) (Gall Bladder's Hollow)

- Cools the Gall Bladder and Liver from Damp-Heat.
- Benefits the diaphragm and chest.
- Tonifies deficiency.

Bl20 Pi Shu (Sp) (Spleen's Hollow)

- Tonifies the Middle Jiao.
- Regulates Sp and tonifies Qi and Blood.
- Strengthens Sp function of transformation and transportation.

Note: Bl17, Bl18 and Bl20 can be combined as a sort of tonic.

Bl21 Wei Shu (St) (Stomach's Hollow)

- Regulates St Qi, transforms dampness.
- Reduces stagnation.
- Not much tonifying.

Bl22 San Jiao Shu (TH) (Triple Burner's Hollow)

● Benefits the water circulation.

Bl23 Shen Shu (Ki) (Kidney's Hollow)

● Tonifies Yin and Yang, benefits Jing, warms the Lower Jiao.
● Supports Yuan Qi.
● Transforms Dampness.
● Strengthens back and spine.
● Benefits the eyes, benefits the ears.
● Nourishes the Water, strengthens the Fire.

Bl24 Qihai Shu (Sea of Qi Hollow)

● Adjusts Qi and Blood.
● Strengthens low back and knees.

Bl25 Da Chang Shu (LI) (Large Intestine's Hollow)

● Frequent use: acute and chronic low back strain.
● Strengthens low back, thighs and knees.
● Regulates intestines and St Qi.
● Transforms stagnation: constipation, diarrhoea.

Bl27 Xiao Chang Shu (SI) (Small Intestine's Hollow)

● Adjusts and moves the Small Intestine.
● Resolves Damp, promotes urination, clears Heat.
● Regulates the Colon.

Bl28 Pang Guan Shu (Bl) (Bladder's Hollow)

● Benefits back and spine.
● Tonifies Yuan Qi.
● Adjusts the Bladder.
● Moves and benefits the water channels.

Bl43 Gaohuang Shu (Vital's Hollow)

● Tonifies the Lungs, strengthens the Spleen, eliminates exhaustion.
● Quietens the Heart.
● Supports Ki Yin and Yang; strengthens Yuan Qi.
● For nocturnal emissions and after illness.
● Needle – Yang Xu.
● Moxa – Yin Xu.

Front Mu points

CV17 Shanzhong (Pe) (Penetrating Odour)

- Not used much to treat the Pericardium – used more as the meeting point of Qi.
- 'Descends the Opposition' – cough and vomiting (Qi going up).
- Opens the chest, stagnation of blood.
- Transforms phlegm, clears diaphragm, clears Lu, quietens cough.
- Don't needle too deeply or too strongly.

CV14 Ju Que (Ht) (Great Palace)

- Affects the whole of the chest.
- Clears the Ht, quietens the spirit, regulates chest and diaphragm.
- Transforms damp stagnation in the middle jiao.
- Symptoms – coughing, Qi rising, painful chest, cardiac pain, palpitations.
- Used a lot for Ht disease and lung stagnation.
- Get needle sensation towards Ht or Lu, needle inwards and upwards.

CV12 Zhong Wan (St) (Middle Cavity)

- Harmonizes St Qi, benefits the St, regulates Qi, benefits the diaphragm.
- Regulates the middle jiao.
- Adjusts ascending and descending functions.
- Transforms mucus.

CV5 Shi Men (TH) (Stone Door)

- Not a main point.
- Some of the books say avoid this point in women because it might cause infertility.

CV4 Guan Yuan (SI) (Hinge at the Source)

- To prevent illness and for tonifying the whole body.
- Supports the Ki, 'firms the foundation' and tonifies Qi.
- Expels cold and damp in SI.
- Separates the clear and turbid.

CV3 Zhong Ji (Bl) (Middle Summit)

- Benefits the Bladder.
- Clears Damp-Heat.

- Tonifies Blood in the uterus, warms the Jing and the uterus.
- Promotes the transformation function of the Bladder.
- Tonifies the Kidney.

Lu1 Zhong Fu (Lu) (Central Residence)

- Used especially for Full conditions, phlegm in the Lu, fierce coughing.
- Circulates and adjusts the Lu Qi.
- Disperses and makes things move.
- Clears excess.

Liv14 Qi Men (Liv) (Expectation's Door)

- Promotes the function of the Liver.
- Regulates the Qi, moves the Blood, transforms congealed Blood.
- Eliminates the retention of food.
- For all female troubles, especially for stoppage of menses.

GB24 Ri Yue (GB) (Sun Moon)

- Promotes the function of GB and Liv.
- Relieves hypochondriac pain.
- Transforms Damp-Heat, harmonizes the Middle Jiao.
- Used for Gallstones.

Liv13 Zhang Men (Sp) (System's Door)

- Promotes the function of the liver, strengthens the spleen.
- Resolves Damp, regulates Qi.
- 'Lumps and bumps in chest and abdomen'.

GB25 Jing Men (Ki) (Capital's Door)

- Used a lot for Kidney stones and inflammation, Damp-Heat and acute pain.
- Warms cold Ki.
- Leads the water to the Bladder.

St25 Tian Shu (LI) (Heaven's Axis)

- Adjusts intestines, especially for diarrhoea and/or constipation.
- Regulates Qi.
- Relieves stagnation of food.
- In menstrual conditions – stagnation of Qi and Blood, dysmenorrhoea.

Lower Ho points of the six Fu

St37 Shang Ju Xu (LI) (Upper Void)

- Most important of the Ho points.
- Treats the Colon organ.
- Dispels the retention of food, cools Damp-Heat, regulates the St and intestines.
- Used in appendicitis.

St39 Xia Ju Shu (SI) (Lower Void)

- Adjusts St and intestines, cools Damp-Heat.
- Used for constipation and diarrhoea.

The other Ho points are:

St36 Zu San Li (St) (Three Measures on the Leg).
Bl40 Wei Zhong (Bl) (Commission the Middle).
Bl39 Wei Yang (TH) (Commission the Yang).
GB34 Yang Ling Quan (GB) (Yang Tomb Spring).

Hui (meeting) points (influential points)

These are important points and all are used frequently. They tend to be added into the prescriptions and the points are chosen on the basis of differentiation of syndromes and added on the base of level or tissue involved. They seem to affect and benefit the Zang/Fu, Blood and Qi.

Liv13 Zhang Men (Zang Organs) (System's Door)

- Benefits all the Zang.
- Benefits the Sp, benefits the Liv.

CV12 Zhong Wan (Fu Organs) (Middle Cavity)

- Used a lot.
- Is the meeting point of all the Fu.
- Borborygmus, vomiting, diarrhoea.

CV17 Shan Zhong (Qi) (Penetrating Odour)

- Meeting point of Qi.

Bl17 Ge Shu (Blood) (Diaphragm's Hollow)

- Meeting point of the diaphragm.
- Most important for the Blood.
- In all blood situations – stuck, deficient, etc. – this point can be added in.
- Vomiting of blood, wasting or consumptive disease.
- Stuck blood due to accident, internal haemorrhage.

GB34 Yang Ling Quan (Tendons) (Yang Tomb Spring)

- For all tendons in the body.

Lu9 Tai Yuan (Arteries) (Great Abyss)

- Arteries and vessels.
- Its true meaning is uncertain, but is likely to be deficiency of vital Qi giving a weak pulse.
- Most important is its use as the Yuan point of the Lu channel.

Bl11 Da Shu (Bone) (Big Shuttle)

- All bone diseases, painful joints and rheumatism, bony Bi and arthritis.
- Osteoporosis, wasting of bones.

GB39 Xuan Zhong (Marrow) (Suspended Time)

- Used to prevent stroke – marrow nourishes the brain – high blood pressure.

3

The Eight Principles

Before considering the emphasis to be placed on the foregoing considerations when it comes to the selection of points for actual treatment, we must now turn to what might be termed an almost alternative approach, i.e. that approach which mainland China now calls Traditional Chinese Medicine, based on the concept of the 'Eight Principles' or 'Eight Approaches' mentioned in the Introduction.

The eight principles are four pairs of contradictory groups of symptoms which are the basic analytical components for differential diagnosis. Location, nature, physical status and stages of an illness are considered.

The four pairs of entities are:

1 Internal (Li)/External (Biao).
2 Cold (Han)/Hot (Jeh).
3 Empty (Xu)/Full (Shi) – deficiency and excess.
4 Yin/Yang – dynamic balance.

Li/Biao (Internal/External)

This pair of entities denotes the depth and location of the symptom complex. External symptoms are projected to the surface of the body, internal symptoms are the manifestations of the abnormal functions of the internal organs. It is sometimes considered to refer also to chronic and acute (True and False) diseases, but this is not necessarily so.

External diseases are often the early stages of the result of exposure to chills etc., and are usually characterized by rapid onset (typical of Wind disease) and can be either muscular, etc. (leading to the so-called Bi syndrome of rheumatic and arthritic disturbances) or in the form of 'chills', with intolerance of cold, mild fever, headaches, aches in the body, nasal obstruction, etc. from some exogenic factor.

External diseases can be associated with either cold or heat, or deficiency (Xu) or excess (Shi). The disease may start externally and progress deeper, and the practitioner must be on the look-out for this, the typical progressions being either through the six jiaos (Tai Yang, Shao

Yang, Yang Ming, Tai Yin, Jue Yin, Shao Yin) or through the so-called Four Radicals (or stages) of energy (Wei, Mixed Wei and Yong, Yong, Blood) or through Heaven, Earth and Man (or the Upper, Middle and Lower Heaters) leading to the involvement of the Zang/Fu organs.

The typical case caused by 'Wind' may, as in all Wind diseases, be combined with either Wind and Cold, Wind and Damp, etc. As we have seen, most illnesses caused by either Wind and/or Cold will give a dislike of those specific entities. It is a superficial condition and the pulse will be correspondingly superficial, whilst the tongue will have either no fur or a thin, whitish fur.

For all external conditions the practitioner must not forget to consider the use of the Tendino-Muscular meridians, but also remember the specific action of the Ching points, also the necessity for getting the Qi and Blood moving, and to use Moxa in cold conditions where Cold and Cold-Damp predominate.

The Wind/Heat conditions are usually similar to local infections, such as acute rhinitis, sinusitis, bronchitis, urticaria, etc., and give the typical acute onsets with fever, inflammation, possible itching in skin conditions, etc., and we would dispel the Wind and Heat using the Lung, Colon and Stomach meridians, with local and distant points such as LI4, LI11, Lu11, St9 and St44.

Repeated exposures to cold and damp can give rise to the 'Bi' syndromes mentioned earlier, and the external type must be differentiated from the internal Bi syndromes where the organs are implicated (usually Ki deficiency).

● Wind Bi causes 'flitting' pains, moving from joint to joint and never settling.
● Cold Bi would give a stagnant effect, with biting pains in the joints.
● Damp Bi is altogether stickier, and causes stiffness.
● There is also a Febrile Bi, which is more constitutional, with redness, pain and swelling in the joints and possible feverishness. This is caused by either Wind-Cold-Damp turning into heat in the body or through attack of Damp-Heat.

Internal (Li) diseases denote a progression of hot illness into the interior of the body, as manifested by high fever and where:

● Ht is involved – restlessness, mental dullness, delirium.
● Liv is involved – convulsions, opisthotonos.
● St is involved – vomiting, abdominal distension, epigastric tenderness.
● Lu is involved – cough, dyspnoea, flaring of nostrils.
● Sp and bowels are involved – diarrhoea, constipation, dysentery.

Interior symptoms are mostly severe and deep, as the pathogenic factors are damaging the Zang/Fu organs.

Internal heat will usually give perspiration, great thirst, bloodshot eyes, rapid pulse, red tongue with a yellow coat (sometimes a reddish-purple tongue) and there is often constipation.

Internal cold – the patient feels chilly with cold extremities, night sweats, loose stools, and a slow and sunken pulse.

Cold/Hot (Han/Jeh)

This is not a measurement of body temperature, but serves to differentiate the nature of the disease. Treatment depends on the differentiation.

Cold entity comes from diminished function or decreased energy and metabolism or decreased resistance. In general, the patient feels cold, is worse in Winter and on cold days, is better for heat and warm foods and drink, has a pale face, clear urine, watery stool, pale tongue with whitish fur, and a slow pulse.

Hot entity comes from general hyperfunction, increase of energy and metabolism and over-reaction to pathogenic factors, and from either external causes such as heatstroke, or from internal ones such as excess of alcohol, hot spicy foods, or anger or other emotions. In general, feels the heat, prefers cooler weather, perspires easily when hot, likes cold food and drinks, has a flushed face, with thirst and a dry mouth, is constipated, and has dark scanty urine, a red tongue with yellowish or brownish fur, whilst the pulse is big, full, fast and gliding.

However, Hot and Cold diseases may be:

- Internal or external origin.
- Internal or external location.
- Shi or Xu (Full or Empty).

Internal cold frequently comes from too much cold food and drink, which can weaken the Yang Qi and cause Xu cold symptoms such as chronic cold diarrhoea. In other cases it can retard the circulation of Qi and Blood and cause Shi cold symptoms with stagnation in the abdomen, giving constipation, abdominal and menstrual pain. The pulse in the Shi type will be slow, firm and tight, and the tongue may be pale and moist. If there is stagnant Qi and Blood the tongue may be purplish. Fur would be thick and white or, if severe, wet and black.

Treatment would be to tonify and warm in the Xu type, and disperse and warm in the Shi type.

Lu, Cold

Lungs are connected to external skin, therefore easily affected by cold.

- Breathless, coughing with thin white mucus, worse lying down (allows Lu Qi and mucus to rise), nasal obstruction, chilliness, general oedema.
- Pulse – slow, slippery and full.
- Tongue – thick, white fur.

Lu, Hot

- Fever, malar flush, sore throat, dyspnoea, cough with thick yellow mucus, pain in chest, dry mouth, thirst, constipation, reddish urine.
- Pulse – fast, overflowing, strong.
- Tongue – either whole tongue or tip red.

LI, Cold

Mainly diarrhoea.

LI, Hot with Dry-Heat:

- Constipation, mouth and lips dry, abdominal distension, breath foul or bitter taste in mouth, dark scanty urine.
- Pulse – rapid, slippery and full.
- Tongue – red with dry, yellow fur.

Li, Hot with Damp-Heat:

- Fever and thirst, abdomen painful, frequent loose stools with offensive odour, mucus and blood in stools, burning in anus, dark scanty urine.
- Pulse – rapid and slippery.
- Tongue – red with greasy, yellow fur.

St, Cold

Either from external factors or too much cold or raw food causing stagnation of St Qi.

- Heartburn and water-brash, sensation of fullness with dull pains and swelling in epigastrium, vomiting of clear fluid, worse with cold or cold food.
- Pulse – slow and fine.
- Tongue – greasy, white fur.

St, Cold-Damp

- Abdominal distension, lack of appetite, body and head feel heavy, tiredness, sweet sticky taste in mouth, loose stool, chronic diarrhoea.
- Pulse – slow, slippery and fine.
- Tongue – greasy, white fur.

St, Heat

From excessive hot, greasy or spicy food or alcohol, or from attack by Liv Fire.

- Dry mouth, burning pain in epigastrium, always hungry, sour vomit of undigested food, foul smell from mouth, bleeding and swollen gums, possible constipation (St heat moves to LI).
- Pulse – rapid, large and slippery.
- Tongue – dry with red body, thick yellow/brown fur.

Sp, Cold-Damp

From either external or internal causes.

- Same symptoms as St, Cold-Damp.

Sp, Heat-Damp

From either external or internal causes. Damp-Heat in the Sp can obstruct the flow of bile in the GB.

- Heaviness in chest and body, lack of appetite, fever, bitter taste in mouth, swelling in ribs and sides, intermittent abdominal pain, hot dysentery, vomiting, red lips, red face, swollen and bloated or face and eyes yellow, scanty dark urine.
- Pulse – rapid and slippery.
- Tongue – greasy, yellow fur.

Ht, Heat

Usually of mental/emotional origin causing the Qi to become 'stuck' and therefore heated, or from an invasion of Liv fire.

- Red face, dry mouth with bitter taste, painful eyes, haemoptysis, haematemesis, irritability, delirium, laughs and talks a lot, insomnia, feeling of heat in chest, urine is hot and deep yellow.
- Pulse – rapid and full.
- Tongue – tip or whole tongue red, dry yellow fur, inflammation or ulceration of tongue or mouth.

Pe, Usually Damp-Heat from mucus (Tanyin)

As with the heart, is usually from a mental/emotional cause or from infection. The first cause will lead to depression and dullness of mind.

- Feverishness, delirium, hyperactivity, dribbling, depression, mania, loss of consciousness.
- Pulse – rapid and slippery.
- Tongue – thick, greasy, yellow fur.

SI, Usually Damp-Heat

If from the Heart could be accompanied by the Ht hot symptoms of pain and ulceration of mouth and tongue.

- Abdominal distension relieved by passing flatus or belching, abdominal pain radiating to spine and testes, pains in penis, retraction of testes, painful dark urination.
- Pulse – rapid and slippery.
- Tongue – tip and sides red, thick yellow fur.

Bl, Damp-Heat

- Fever; dry mouth; pain in lumbar region; frequency with hot burning painful urination; scanty dark-red or turbid urine with abnormal smell; urinary incontinence with severe pain and thick bloody urine.
- Pulse – rapid, slippery and wiry.
- Tongue – red body, greasy yellow fur.

GB, Damp-Heat

From either infection, the Liver, chronic excess of rich food or alcohol.

- Pain in thorax and flanks; dull sensation in stomach; bitter taste in mouth; bitter vomit; restless, disturbed sleep; irritability; blurred vision; transient deafness; possible jaundice; scanty dark urine; alternating chills and fevers.
- Pulse – rapid, slippery and wiry.
- Tongue – sides red, greasy yellow fur.

Liv, Cold

- If in the Liv meridian, leads either to hydrocele or to retraction of scrotum and testes.
- Pulse – slow, deep and wiry.

Li, Hot

From either chronic 'sticking' of Qi (usually emotional), or from too much rich food.

- Head feels swollen, violent headache; sudden deafness or tinnitus; red, swollen eyes, lacrimation; dry mouth, bitter taste in mouth; haemoptysis; sour bitter vomit; depressed and irritable; restless sleep; pain in ribs and sides; spasms and twitching; constipated with dry stool.
- Pulse – rapid, full and wiry.
- Tongue – red body and sides, yellow fur.

Empty/Full (Xu/Shi)

'Signify the course of the body struggling against the noxious pathogenic factors, and the variation in the strength of the body's reactions' (Lee and Cheung, 1978).

In deficiency the vital energy is drained, co-ordination of Yin and Yang is impaired and there is general hypofunction and lack of vitality and resistance.

In excess there is an excess of noxious Qi, which includes both the strength of the external pathogenic factors and the resistance of the reaction of the body, i.e. a severe struggle is still going on. If the body's resistance is weak but the pathogenic factor is still strong, then there will be a picture of mixed Shi and Xu.

Xu disease

This is characterized by weakness, with an empty pulse, possibly a thick, tender tongue with little or no fur, and pains which will tend to be dull and aching and better for massage and pressure.

Emptiness of Qi is usually associated with the Lungs, although LI, St, Sp, Ht and Ki can also be affected. It manifests as a pale face, lack of vitality, timidity, excess nervous perspiration in daytime, lack of appetite, dizziness and palpitations, and sometimes dyspnoea. The pulse is empty, short and fine, whilst the tongue tends to be large and flabby, slightly pale, with no fur.

Emptiness of Yang can come from a constitutional weakness, bad eating habits, over-work, over-indulgence or just old age. There is a weakness of warming energies which produces cold symptoms, this therefore being termed empty-cold. It is especially associated with a weakness of Ki Yang, although Sp may also be affected. As well as the usual signs of empty Qi there will be a general dislike of cold, a cold feeling in the body, watery stool, copious clear urine, and a pale or greyish face. The pulse will be empty, but may also be slow and deep or weak and fine. The tongue will be pale and damp with a thin, white fur.

Lu

Said to suffer from empty Qi but not empty Yang. Will get the usual signs and symptoms of a Xu condition, but can also get a dry skin, stuttering, catching cold easily due to a weakness of Wei energy, excess urination, general feeling of cold, cough and asthma.

LI

Usually the empty and cold symptoms originate from empty cold in the Sp, but prolonged damp heat in the LI can weaken its Qi energy, to produce chronic diarrhoea, prolapse of the rectum, a feeling of abdominal discomfort and possible shivering.

St/Sp

Weakness of the Qi will give poor transformation of food and drink producing symptoms of weak digestion. The most likely causes are poor food intake, or possibly too much cold food and drink, which will dampen the Sp Fire. Symptoms could include a sallow face, loose watery stools with undigested food, oedema, tiredness, lack of appetite, belching, abdominal or thoracic discomfort, and rectal or uterine prolapse. With a deficiency of Sp Yang one could also find general coldness in the limbs, abdominal distension, nausea and vomiting, cachexia and chronic haemorrhages.

Ht

Usually from either emotional causes, or weakness after a long illness. Empty Qi gives palpitations and breathlessness, pallor and anxiety. Empty Yang will add a greyish pale face, cardiac oedema, confusion, coldness, and profuse sweating. The pulse in both cases will feel knotted, but with empty Qi it will tend to be intermittent whilst with empty Yang it will be slow and minute.

Ki

Emptiness is usually constitutional or from some debilitating factor. Empty Ki Qi will not hold the fluids, therefore one will get frequent pale urination, dribbling after urination, incontinence, nocturnal emissions, weakened libido, premature ejaculation, infertility and vaginal discharges, and as the Ki fails to hold down the Lu Qi, one can get dyspnoea and asthma. There can also be the usual Ki symptom of pains in the lumbar area and knees, also tinnitus and vertigo.

When Yang is also deficient the lumbar area will be aching and cold, there will be pains in the knees, etc., chilliness, impotence, oliguria, oedema (especially of the lower limbs) and diarrhoea in the early morning. If severe, the tongue may be wet and blackish.

Apart from symptoms of emptiness in the organs, one can also have emptiness in the **Blood**. Blood depends primarily upon diet, then on the functions of the Ki and St/Sp energies which are responsible for its formation. It is moved around the body by the Qi, therefore stagnation of Qi can lead to stagnation of Blood. (Conversely, the formation of Qi depends upon the nourishment brought by the Blood.)

Empty Blood symptoms are general pallor, dry falling hair, cold limbs and a general 'dryness' – encompassing the stool, mouth, scanty urine, amenorrhoea, etc. The pulse is thin, choppy and hollow, and the tongue is pale with no fur.

One can also have the condition of **Empty Yin** (Yin Xu). When the Yin is deficient it will no longer be able to cool and moisten efficiently and the Yang Qi will tend to float upwards giving rise to symptoms of **Empty Heat**. Yin Xu is caused mainly by a deficiency of Ki Yin.

Empty heat will give a slight feverishness in the afternoon, also sores in the mouth and sore throat. The rising Yang will lead to insomnia, irritability, spots before the eyes and vertigo, and also general debility from the weakness of Yin. This latter will manifest as a general dryness – as we saw with empty blood – but there will also be night sweats because the Wei Qi (which should be deeper at night) will tend to float to the surface and open the pores. This loss of fluid and of Wei Qi will lead to loss of weight and to emaciation. The pulse will be thin, empty and floating, the tongue bright red and dry, with no fur.

Shi diseases are often regarded as the more acute stage – traditionally characterized by a flushed face, good spirits, loud voice and forceful protrusion of the tongue!

Apart from a fullness of Cold and Heat, which have already been covered, there can also be fullness of Damp, Mucus, Damp-Heat, Stagnant Qi, Stagnant Blood and Stagnant Food.

Damp:

- Caused by exposure to damp, or by diet.
- Is stagnant, heavy, sticky and greasy.

- Stagnates in head, chest, abdomen and limbs.
- Poor transformation of food in St/Sp gives rise to indigestion and fluid retention, with such symptoms as nausea, vomiting, loose stools, scanty urination, oedema, lack of thirst, heavy head and limbs, sweet sticky taste in mouth, vertigo and exudatory skin disorders.
- The pulse is slow, slippery and fine, the tongue coated with thick white or dirty yellow fur.

Mucus (Tanyin):

- Is rather similar to damp and is usually caused by poor function of St/Sp caused by faulty diet – too much greasy food, etc.
- It can be of either a hot or a cold nature.
- If it affects the Lu it will give cough or asthma with heavy phlegm, blocked nose, etc. In the Ht it will block the free passage of Shen and cause hysteria, mania, fits, fever or possibly coma.
- If it blocks the St it will cause gastritis, nausea and vomiting.
- Tanyin can also block the superficial meridians, to cause numbness, hemiplegia or deviation of eyes and mouth, or can block the skin to cause soft, movable nodules.
- The pulse is usually slippery and wiry, the tongue covered with thick, greasy, dirty fur.

Damp-Heat:

- Either externally from a hot, steamy climate or from an accumulation of damp in patients with a 'hot' internal energy. The heat will make the sticky watery discharges of damp more painful, purulent and urgent.
- It usually occurs in warm, damp areas of the body such as the genitalia or the bowels. In the genitalia it will produce itching and irritation, purulent discharges, etc. In the bowels it will produce painful, urgent, foul-smelling stools, possibly containing mucus or blood.
- The pulse is slippery and rapid, the tongue red, with a greasy yellow fur.

Stagnant Qi:

- Usually caused by Liv dysfunction and due to bowel blockage, accumulation of Qi gas in the abdomen or emotional disturbance.
- Symptoms are congestion in trunk or abdomen, soreness, distension and a bloated feeling.
- The blockages are palpable but tend to move around and are usually better with belching, flatus, etc.
- Worse when emotionally disturbed.

Stagnant Blood:

- Caused by local trauma, cold or stagnant Qi (Qi moves the blood).
- Symptoms are localized pain (sharp, stabbing), intermittent haemorrhages, clots in blood, possible cyanosis, capillary congestion.
- Lumps are hard and fixed.
- Menses are absent or delayed, scanty, dark, clotted. Premenstrual tension.
- The pulse is deep, full and firm, and the tongue can be dark purple.

Stagnant Food:

- Caused by excessive or irregular eating, causing the St Qi to rebel upwards.
- No appetite, congestion in chest, abdominal distension, belching, water brash, vomiting.
- Pulse full and slippery, tongue coated with thick, greasy fur.

Yin/Yang

This is the basic, underlying classification. The general qualities of Yin and Yang are already known, and are summarized below.

Yin diseases are characterized by deficiency; cold hypoactivity; paleness; liking for warmth; constipation, which is stagnant and inactive, or diarrhoea, with a watery stool and no pain or smell; copious clear urine with no smell; a slow, weak or sunken pulse; and a pale tongue with a thin, white coating.

Yang diseases are mostly acute, hot and superficial. The patient is flushed and restless, likes the cold, and is talkative with loud, coarse breathing. Constipation is accompanied by heat and discomfort; diarrhoea by urgency and a foul smell. The urine is concentrated and foul smelling. The pulse tends to be rapid and thready; the tongue red with a heavier coating.

The other symptoms of Internal/External, Cold/Hot and Empty/Full are superimposed over and included under the Yin/Yang basic diagnosis and will modify the symptom picture.

Generally, in a Yin disease one would tonify the Yang and/or disperse the Yin. In a Yang disease one would disperse the Yang and/or tonify the Yin.

4

The rules of acupuncture

So far we have looked at the three fundamental approaches to the practice of acupuncture – the Five Elements, the use of Antique points and the Eight Approaches. These three are taken into account in all our basic diagnoses. The Five Elements diagnosis is founded on an overall assessment to decide into which element category the patient may be classified, and in this context it is the pulses which should (at least in theory) provide the decisive answer. I have said 'in theory' because in practice most practitioners find great difficulty in arriving at a conclusive picture, and in any case the actual 'reading' is extremely subjective – five different practitioners often arriving at five different answers. A further source of difficulty is that in these enlightened times the majority of our patients consult us only after having unsuccessfully run the gamut of various other modalities, and are usually in the process of taking regular drugs which successfully mask any pulse picture upon which we could rely. My own feeling is that practitioners should beware of looking too hard to find an imbalance – if a genuine one exists they won't have to look for it, it will be self-evident, whilst other aspects of diagnosis, such as skin colour, typology and mannerisms, will also augment what the pulses tell us.

Having been informed of the element involved using the Five Element approach, the Traditional Chinese Medicine (TCM) approach will now tell us further as to the type of involvement – hot or cold, internal or external. Consideration of the Welling Theory is inevitably bound up with what, for want of a better title, we call the 'Rules of Acupuncture', or the ways in which we select and apply the appropriate points. Some authorities quote nine rules, others quote ten – in reality it doesn't matter because practitioners add rules of their own as their experience increases, but for the sake of simplicity I'll give the ones which I consider important and then go into them in detail:

1 Ah Shi points
2 Local points
3 End and distal points
4 Local and distant points

 5 Points with special action
 6 Key points (of the Eight Extra meridians)
 7 Five Element points
 8 Shu and Mu points
 9 Formulae
10 Points in opposition
11 Points in line
12 Pathogenic relationships (e.g. GB21 to expel Wind in stiff neck)

1. Ah Shi points

I never cease from repeating that the main trouble with acupuncture, at least insofar as the serious practitioner is concerned, is that even bad acupuncture works, and this holds true to a very great extent where some of our more 'scientific' brethren are involved. Steadfastly refusing to admit the evidence of 5000 years of successful achievement in the treatment of internal as well as external conditions, they unite in refusing to acknowledge the very existence of the meridians, and dismiss as medieval nonsense the idea of Yin and Yang or of Qi energy. But they also unite in agreeing that if you stick the needle in where it hurts you often get amazing results! The thing is, of course, that if one has any blockage in the energy flow it will often manifest as a painful nodule or fibrotic locus in the muscle fibres – this may arise from a purely local condition or it may even be a viscero-somatic reflex from a deeper pathology, but a needle judiciously inserted and manipulated will disperse the blockage and thus remove the symptom. This approach is lauded by Dr Baldry in his book *Acupuncture, Trigger Points and Musculoskeletal Pain* (1989), but is greatly extended by Mark Seem in *A New American Acupuncture* (1993). Mark Seem has the advantage of a deep understanding of TCM and other acupuncture schools and theories (his *Acupuncture Energetics* is strongly recommended) and his system of myofascial release is a truly fascinating concept.

As I have said, an energy blockage may result in the production of a local area of painful fibrosis or muscle spasm, but careful palpation of the abdomen over the front Mu points or lateral to the spine over the back Shu points can also demonstrate painful areas. These are extremely useful in diagnosis as the position and type of pain, and whether elicited on superficial or deep pressure, etc., can not only tell us the possible Zang/Fu involved but also the underlying condition – Yin or Yang, Hot or Cold, Full or Empty.

One common source of argument amongst acupuncturists is whether one should first treat the acute presenting symptoms (the Biao) or the underlying cause (the Ben). Lavier (a leading figure in the introduction of acupuncture to the UK and translator of Wu Wei Ping's work in Taiwan) always used to say treat the acute symptoms first because they will often mask the deeper cause – once these have been dealt with then treat the basic systemic condition to prevent them from recurring. This is presenting a somewhat simplistic view and does depend purely upon an assessment of the situation.

The old Chinese saying 'Where the pain is, there is the point' is almost 100 per cent true, but the question should be asked 'Is it referred, and if so, from where?' We have both viscero-somatic reflexes and somatico-visceral ones. In the former the use of an Ah Shi point can remove a local pain but will rarely affect the Zang/Fu disturbance. In the latter, the secondary effect upon the viscera can produce an improvement in general well-being but might well need more local work (or possibly an osteopathic approach) to effect a cure.

2. Local points

These are not necessarily the same as the Ah Shi points, although they frequently exhibit this characteristic. Ah Shi points are not always recognized acupuncture points, but 'local points' always are, being exactly what their name implies – points in the area of the body which is presenting the trouble. Examples are Bitong or LI20 for nasal problems, TH4 for the wrist, and CV12 for the stomach (disregarding the fact that this is also a Mu point). Some treatments can consist almost exclusively of local points, such as LI15, Jianneiling, Naoshang and SI10 for capsulitis of the shoulder. In other cases the local points are added in almost as extras to more strongly working distant points.

3. End and distal points

This is the use of a specific technique of opposite action on near and distant points. If the trouble is at one end of a meridian one takes the appropriate action on the point of the meridian concerned and the opposite action on the point at its far end, the Tsing point. For example, if there is inflammation or overactivity at the internal canthus, one drains Bl1 and then stimulates Bl67. If there were underactivity in the eye, one would stimulate Bl1 then drain Bl67. If the trouble is not at the extreme end of the meridian the appropriate action is taken on the concerned point and the opposite action upon the Ho point of the meridian; for example, with trouble in the region of St3, drain here and then stimulate St36, or for spasm in the lumbar area drain Bl24 then stimulate Bl40 (Weizhong). An interesting extension of this technique is to add a further manipulation to the distant point by repeating the similar action to that used on the local point after having used the above manipulation; for example, for overaction in the Bl24 area drain Bl24 then stimulate Bl40, which is then immediately drained without removing the needle. This technique, known as Long Hu Chiao Chan (the Battle of the Tiger and the Dragon), is actually a relatively advanced manipulation done over a period of five of the patient's respiratory cycles and has to be demonstrated to be learnt properly.

4. Local and distant points

Strangely enough, this is *not* the same as the preceding rule. The basic principle of treatment is that in acute conditions we use a stronger action upon distant points than upon local ones, whilst in chronic conditions the reverse holds true, with a greater emphasis being placed upon the local points. When one has been in practice long enough to be able to 'tune in' to what the patient is feeling and how their body is behaving, one will be able to appreciate the reason for this. In acute conditions there may be so much local reaction, the local energy is so perturbed that too much interference could exacerbate the condition – one approaches the local site with caution and works rather by drawing the energy away down the meridian. (A hypofunction is less likely to have locally acute symptoms unless of traumatic origin and one stimulates the energy supplying the area, again by the use of remote points.) In a chronic condition, however, the local malfunction has become deep and fixed and needs a strong attack – one hits hard locally and supports it by appropriate action on the meridial energy. (Note that we are taking a *similar* action on the distant point and not a dissimilar one as in Rule 3.)

This rule usually implies the use of distant points on the same meridian as the major meridian for the affected area, but this is not invariably the case, and one usually uses points which are known to have a strong effect upon the area generally, i.e. GB20 as a local point and for its specific effect upon 'Wind in the Head' (see Rule 12, Pathogenic Relations) with GB40 as a distant point, or sciatica using Huanchung as a local point and Bl60 as a distant point.

Included in this rule we might also bring in the use of adjacent points which are midway between local and remote. Table 4.1 gives a brief summary of the more commonly used points for the various areas.

A further adjacent study to 'local and distant' points are the two related concepts of 'origins and ends' and 'roots and branches' (not to be confused with the Branches of the Celestial Stems). The two are

Table 4.1

Diseased area	Remote points		Adjacent points	Local points
	Upper limb	Lower limb		
Face and forehead	LI3	St43	GV20	GV23
Head and temple	TH5	GB43	GB20	Taiyang, GB8
Nape	SI3	BL66	Bl11	GV16, GB20
Eye	SI6	GB37	GV23	Bl1, TH23
Nose	LI11	St45	Bl7	LI20, LI19
Mouth and cheek	LI4	St44	SI17	St4, St6
Ear	TH3	GB41	SI17	GB2, TH17
Throat	Lu11	Ki6	GV15	CV23, CV22
Chest	Lu5	St40	St19	CV17
Costal region	TH6	GB34	Bl18	Sp17, Liv14
Hypochondrium		GB38	Liv14	GB26, GB27
Upper abdomen	Pe6	St36	CV16	CV12
Lower abdomen		Sp6	St25	CV4
Lumbar area	SI6	Bl40	GB25	BL18, Bl23
Rectum		Bl57	Bl30	GV1, Bl35

Table 4.2 Roots and Branches

	Origin	End	Root area	Branch area
Lu	Lu11	Lu1 area	Radial pulse, Lu9	Area of axillary artery, Lu1
LI	LI1	LI20 area	Cubital fossa, LI11, LI14	Cheek and mandible, LI20, CV24
St	St45	St4	Lateral second toe, St45	Frontal face, St9, St4
Sp	Sp1	Upper abdomen	3 cun above internal maleolus, Sp6	Back Shi point root of tongue, Bl20, CV23
Ht	Ht9	Axilla	Ulnar side of wrist, Ht7	Back Shu point, Bl15
SI	SI1	SI18	Above outer wrist, SI6	1 cun above eye, Bl2, Yuyao
Bl	Bl67	Bl1	5 cun above heel, Bl59	Eye, Bl1
Ki	Ki1	CV23	2 cun below internal malleolus, Ki6, Ki2	Back Shu point, Bl23
Pe	Pe9	Chest	Pe6	Pe1
TH	TH1	TH23	TH3	TH19, TH23
GB	GB44	GB2	Between 4/5 metatarsals, GB43, GB44	Front of ear, GB2, SI19
Liv	Liv1	Chest	Liv4 area	Back Shu point, Bl18

nearly the same, yet not quite, for 'origins and ends' relates to the energy in one specific meridian or channel, whilst 'roots and branches' tends to refer more to the circulation of Qi in the body as a whole and therefore covers a wider area, with a more lateral distribution.

An important fact to note is that when we use the term 'end point' in this context we are referring to the point on the body, trunk or head where the Qi flow ends and *not* to the distal end of the channel. The well, or Tsing point, is the origin.

Similarly, the branches are higher and the roots are lower. The Head, Shoulders, Back and Chest are the branches, the roots are the extremities of the limbs below the knees and elbows.

The Tsing points are regarded as the origins because they are the meeting places of Yin and Yang and are the 'grand connections' of life, but whereas in every channel the origin is the Tsing point, the ends are frequently points in the area, whilst with the roots and branches concept the areas subserved are wider still, as shown in Table 4.2.

5. Points with special action

This refers mainly to the Hui or 'influential' points, as given in Chapter 2 on the Antique points:

- Liv13 for the Zang organs
- CV12 for the Fu viscera
- CV17 for Qi and the Respiratory function
- Bl17 for Blood
- GB34 for the Tendons
- Lu9 for Vessels and Pulse
- Bl11 for Bone
- GB39 for Marrow

However, it can also refer to the use of points which have a particularly strong effect upon certain organs or functions, for example Sp6 for all gynaecological conditions and also to affect the three Yin lines of the leg, Sp8 for the uterus, Bl60 for pain generally, St39 for poor circulation in the lower limb, and Bl57 for anal conditions. We must also be careful not to overlook the many non-meridial points – the use of these is *mainly* connected with their special action, such as Dannangxue for gall-bladder problems, or Lanwei for appendicitis. These and many others can be especially important points to bear in mind.

However, it is not only individual points we may find of special use; there are a number of special groups of points which we may also insert under the heading of specific use and amongst the foremost of these are the so-called 'Windows of the Sky'.

The Ling Shu (the second part of the *Nei Ching*, Chapter 21) states 'All the energies Yang come from the Yin (because the Yin is Earth) and the Yin engenders the Yang. These Yang energies always ascend from the lower part of the body towards the head but if they are interrupted in their pathway they cannot climb beyond the abdomen. In that case one must find out which meridian is affected. One tonifies the Yin (as the Yin engenders the Yang) and disperses the Yang so that the energy is attracted towards the top of the body and the circulation is re-established'.

This is part of the basic circulation of the Yang energy, which flows down the tendino-muscular meridians as Wei energy, enters into the principal meridians at the Tsing points and into the deeper circulation at the Ho points, whence it flows up to the head to repeat the cycle.

If a blockage occurs in the cycle, the Windows of the Sky points are used to remove it. Of these there are five main ones, of which four lie on roughly the same line on the neck – St9, LI18, TH16, Bl10 and Lu3 – and their specific symptomatology is as follows:

St9   Severe pain in the head, fullness in the chest, dyspnoea.
LI18   Loss of voice.
TH16   Sudden deafness, blurred vision.
Bl10   Spasms and muscular contractions, fainting, 'feet cannot support him'.
Lu3   Great thirst (from Liv/Lu disharmony), epistaxis, bleeding from mouth.

There are also a further four 'secondary' Windows of the Sky points which can prove useful – GV15, SI16, SI17 and Pe1.

Points of the Four Seas

Another group (or groups) of points of importance are the 'Points of the Four Seas'. The Four Seas are described in Chapter 35 of the Ling Shu. Together they constitute an ensemble which regulates and co-ordinates all the human exchanges.

● The first is the Sea of Energy (the Chest) governed by CV17, St9 and Bl10.
● The second is the Sea of Nourishment (the Stomach) governed by St30 and St36.
● The third is the Sea of Meridians (or Blood) (GV and Chong Mo) governed by Bl11, St37 and St39.
● The fourth is the Sea of Marrow (the Brain) governed by GV16 and GV20.

Sea of Energy

CV17 (Master of the Qi) is situated in the middle of the breast, and regulates the relationship of the breath, respiration, inhalation and exhalation.

St9 is the Window of the Sky point which controls the *ascent* of the Yang of Man towards Heaven.

Bl10 is the Window of the Sky point which controls the *descent* of the Yang of the head towards the body, i.e. the Yang of Heaven downwards to Earth and Man (see Fig. 4.1).

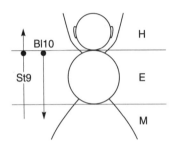

Figure 4.1

The essence of these three points is that of Heaven, with its relationship of breath, air and celestial energy to earthly nourishment and, via its connections with the head and neck, of Heaven and Man.

Sea of Nourishment

St30 controls all the mutations and metabolism of Yang nourishment and also the distribution of Qi throughout the body via the nourishment derived from the food. It is also a point of Chong Mo, which determines its role in this context.

St36, the Ho point, regulates all the bowels (GB, St, SI, LI and Bl), all digestion (complements St30) and the drainage of the lower part of the body (the Earth of Man) via the energy of the blood (contrast with Bl10, which governs the drainage of the upper part).

The essence is Earth, referring to nourishment and the lower part of the body.

Sea of Meridians (or Blood)

Bl11 (the Master Weaver) governs the 'binding' of the whole body, wherein the binding is material in the bones (it is the control point for bones) and immaterial in the meridians (it is the Sea of the Meridians).

It therefore controls the framework upon which life is built and upon which it can thrive and prosper.

St37 governs all movements of Yang towards Yin (corresponds to Autumn).

St39 governs all movements of Yin towards Yang (corresponds to Spring) (see Fig. 4.2).

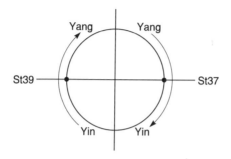

Figure 4.2

These three points therefore govern all exchanges in the interior of the body, with Bl11 governing the basic material and immaterial framework and exchange of Yang to Yin and Yin to Yang via St37 and St39.

Sea of Marrow

GV16 and GV20 from the symptomatology govern all the means of contact with the exterior of the limbs and head, and act like an antenna for the eyes, ears, nose and mouth, the external genitalia, the skin and the mucosa.

The essence is relationship with the Exterior, just as the Sea of the Meridians governs the interior.

The Four Seas therefore form two couples which govern all the exchanges in the body and may be regarded as the seas of Heaven, Earth, Interior and Exterior, with the first couple governing all the exchanges between Heaven and Earth, and the second all those between the Interior and the Exterior.

Symptomatology

Sea of Energy	Full – pain in chest, red face, dyspnoea.
	Empty – Not enough energy to talk.
Sea of Nourishment	Full – abdominal distension.
	Empty – anger, with lack of appetite.

Sea of Meridians	Full – feels as if body enlarged. Empty – as if body shrunk; affected, but cannot say how, and resents it.
Sea of Marrow	Full – light sensations in the body and great strength with a longer life than usual. Empty – whirling sensations in the brain, ringing in ears, fatigued tibia, dizziness, blurred vision, fatigue, love of sleep.

Use

One can think of the use of these points in those cases where one cannot arrive at a precise diagnosis, or in cases which fail to respond to all the usual treatments involving the Eight Principles, organ dysfunction, a principal or secondary meridian, the Five Elements, etc. One should then query if there could be an imbalance between Heaven and Earth or between the Interior and the Exterior.

Examples

Sea of Marrow – The brain is that part of the body which 'reflects' the exterior world to our understanding, and is the controller of our contact with the exterior. Symptoms might present as simultaneous headaches; eye troubles with swollen eyelids; ear, nose and teeth troubles; swelling in the skin, nipples, vulva or penis, hands and feet; joint pains from ligaments and tendons; and symptoms worse at night or in the evening or in bed, when the contacts with the exterior are noticeably diminished.

Sea of Nourishment (of Earth) – as its name implies, this Sea is naturally concerned with the formation and utilization of the Qi and Blood, and its symptomatology will reflect this producing pain and weakness in the lower limbs; chronic digestive troubles with gastric pain; nausea; diarrhoea with undigested food; blood troubles with lipothymea; hypotension; vertigo; respiratory troubles with weak abdominal breathing (lower part of lung). All this would show a weakness in the lower part of the body, most likely associated with a disturbance in the spiritual energy of the Heavens.

As each case is different, each case should be considered on its merits and the Four Seas points augmented with other specific points chosen for the particular case as required.

The Four Seas combinations should be used with discretion – they are powerful points, and misuse could severely aggravate the condition.

6. Key points of the Eight Extra meridians

For a detailed study of these vessels the reader is referred to Low (1983), but the most important fact to be borne in mind about these meridians is that they contain the 'ancestral energy', the Xian Tian Zhi Qi or Pre-Heaven Qi derived from our genetic inheritance. They are considered to act as reservoirs of the energy, supplying the vital essence to depleted meridians as required, but also absorbing any excess for storage for future use. Again we are dealing with a symbolical representation. It is stated that this vital essence is stored in the kidneys and the predominant consideration here is that the ancient Chinese concept of the kidneys and their function is as much or more concerned with the adrenal glands as it is with the mundane Western concept of the kidneys as organs of excretion. The adrenal glands sit on the top of the kidneys in close anatomical relationship, and it is possible that some rudimentary knowledge of the action of the adrenal cortex in producing the corticosteroids gave rise to the statement that 'the Kidneys rule the bones'. Some authorities also consider that Chong Mo (which consists largely of points on the Kidney channel) arises from the adrenal medulla. Suffice it to say that the Eight Extra meridians apparently exert their effect mainly through hormonal and neurological controls, and the use of Bl1 to stimulate the anterior pituitary in the production of somatotrophic and gonadotrophic hormones, combined with the use of the appropriate key points is of great interest. In this context Bl1 is a point of extreme importance, being a reunion point for no less than 10 acupuncture meridians – the principal meridians of St, Bl, SI and TH, the divergent meridians of Sp, Ht, St and SI, and the Yang Chiao and the Yin Chiao. There is also the suggestion of an internal pathway from Du Mo.

One can naturally use the key points, as their name implies, to open up the specific irregular vessel required, but one can also use them for their own individual effect added on to this; for example, SI3 will affect the SI line and is extremely useful as a remote point for cervical problems, but in its role as the key point of Du Mo it will also affect the general Yang of the dorsal and cervical areas. In cases of migraine we frequently work on the GB channel, and the more usual remote point is GB43 (see Table 4.2). However, one might decide it was a case of 'too much above, not enough below' where the energy was concerned, and one might wish to help this by 'loosening the belt' and substituting GB41 to affect Dai Mo. Sp4 is a point frequently added, particularly in female problems, to bring the effect of Chong Mo to bear.

7. Five Element points

The use of these has already been fully described in Chapter 1. They may also be added into a prescription to bring in the Mother/Son effect as required.

8. Shu and Mu points

These are naturally amongst the most frequently used points on the body and form an almost indispensable part of any formula, particularly in the more chronic cases where the organs rather than the meridians are concerned; these latter will be affected only secondarily. Remember the more common usage given earlier – use the Back Shu points for tonifying the Zang organs, which suffer from weakness; use the Front Mu points for affecting the Fu, which tend to suffer from obstruction.

9. Formulae

The use of these is pretty well inescapable. We all say it should never be done and that all acupuncture treatment should be tailored to the individual case at the time of presentation. Of course this is true and we should always do this, but we still fall back upon formulae without realizing it. We use those points which both textbooks and our own experience have taught us are the most effective for dealing with a particular type of case, and we make variations on a basic theme as the various circumstances warrant. Five Element transfer, of course, cannot really come into this category, but TCM Zang/Fu syndromes most definitely do, and the more alternative formulae the practitioners have at their disposal, the better; but *always* with the proviso that they know exactly the action of every point in that formula and why they are using it. The blind use of a formula just because that is what the books say is nothing more or less than quackery.

10. Points in opposition

This refers to the use of points on the opposite side of the body to the one under treatment. Working via the spinal reflex this rule can sometimes augment the treatment, and is sometimes the only viable method. Augmentation is particularly valuable in some cases of hemiplegia where, to quote from my own book on musculoskeletal conditions (Low, 1987), 'if the paralysis is of under three months' duration, reduce the points on the affected side and stimulate those on the unaffected side – in the earlier stages the channels on the affected side are Shi due to stagnation, wind and phlegm, whilst the sound side is relatively Xu, so we must tonify it. If the paralysis is of over three months duration, first reduce the points on the *sound* side and then reinforce the points on the affected side with needle and moxa.'

The points in opposition are the only viable alternatives (apart from scalp needling) in cases of phantom limb, when treatment of the appropriate points on the remaining limb can often produce amazing results.

11. Points in line

This refers simply to the use of consecutive points on the same meridian, and is usually used more for purely local treatment. This can often produce a very strong effect and occasionally, in a weak patient, may cause fainting – so handle with care!

12. Pathogenic relationships

This is the selection of points for their specific effects upon the so-called perverse influences, the 'Spirit of the Points' given in many books on TCM. It is on this basis that all the treatments of modern Chinese acupuncture are based, and a summary is given here:

Lu1	Disperses fullness in the chest.
Lu5	Eliminates Fire in the Lu, calms the ascending Qi.
Lu6	Eliminates Heat, regulates Lu Qi, makes Lu Qi descend, barrier point.
Lu7	Dispels External Wind, strengthens the dispersing function of Lu.
Lu9	Dispels Internal Wind, tonifies Lu Yin and strengthens Lu function; resolves Phlegm.
Lu10	Eliminates Heat from the Lu, eliminates head Fire (Fire point of Lu).
Lu11	Eliminates External Wind-Heat.
LI1	Dispels Penetrating Wind.
LI4	Dispels all Wind, stimulates dispersing function of Lu, stimulates intestines.
LI8	Exit Barrier point.
LI11	Reduces Heat in St and LI, cools Internal Heat and eliminates Wind-Heat.

LI14	Local for arm and shoulder.
LI15	Eliminates Penetrating Wind, entry Barrier point.
LI20	Dispels Wind-Heat, local for nasal blockages.

St2	Dispels External and Internal Wind.
St4	Dispels Wind, stimulates the meridians, helps the joints.
St6	Calms External and Internal Wind, removes blockages in the meridians, removes Heat in the Yang Ming.
St7	Dispels Wind, stimulates the meridians, specific for osteo-chondritis of the mandibular joint.
St8	Dispels Wind, useful for vertigo.
St18	For breast problems, gallstones.
St21	Stimulates function of St and Sp.
St25	Stimulates circulation of Blood and Qi, Mu point of LI.
St28	Eliminates Damp-Heat from Lower Heater.
St29	Moves stagnation of Blood and Qi, useful in dysmenorrhoea.
St31	Stimulates movement of Qi in the legs, entry Barrier point.
St34	Useful where severe pain.
St35	Removes blockage in meridian.
St36	Regulates circulation of Blood and Qi, eliminates Wind and Damp, regulates St and Sp, stimulates the energy.
St37	Too much energy in upper part of body, removes Damp-Heat.
St38	For acute shoulder conditions.
St39	For too little energy in lower part of body, exit Barrier point.
St40	Transforms Dampness, dries up the Sp, resolves Phlegm.
St41	Eliminates Cold-Damp.
St43	Eliminates Wind, cools St.
St44	Removes Fullness in St, blockage in bowels.
St45	Removes Heat in Yang Ming, useful in insomnia.

Sp1	Strengthens Sp function of holding Blood, tonifies Sp.
Sp2	Warms up the Sp (Fire point).
Sp3	Stimulates Sp, removes Internal and External Damp.
Sp4	Balances St and Sp, key point of Chong Mo.
Sp5	Removes Dampness, strengthens St and Sp.
Sp6	Eliminates Damp, stimulates circulation of Blood and Qi, strengthens all Tsu Yin lines.
Sp8	Regulates Blood, adjusts the uterus, entry Barrier point.
Sp9	Removes Damp-Heat from Lower Heater.
Sp10	Dispels Wind, dispels Heat from Blood, regulates circulation of Ying Qi and Blood.

Sp12	Exit Barrier point.
Sp15	Useful in abdominal distension.

Ht3	Regulates Ht Qi.
Ht5	Causes Fire from the head to descend, calms the mind, affects the tongue.
Ht6	Removes Mucus from Ht, exit Barrier point.
Ht7	Calms the Ht, generally sedative.
Ht9	Stimulates Ht Qi.

SI1	Dispels Wind-Heat.
SI3	Eliminates Internal Wind-Heat, key point of Du Mo.
SI4	Disperses Damp-Heat from SI, stimulates Tai Yang.
SI5	Regulates SI Qi, good for Damp-Heat in knees.
SI6	Entry Barrier point.
SI11	Eliminates stagnant Qi from chest, exit Barrier point.
SI18	Dispels Wind.
SI19	Removes obstruction from meridian, clears the ears.

Bl1	Dispels Internal Wind, eliminates Heat.
Bl2	Dispels Wind, calms the Liv.
Bl7	Eliminates Wind from upper part of body.
Bl10	Dispels Wind, stimulates the meridians.
Bl11	Special point for bones.
Bl12	Expels Wind, helps circulation of Qi and strengthens the dispersing function of the Lu.
Bl13	Dispels Heat from the Lu and helps their dispersing function.
Bl15	Stimulates circulation of Qi and Blood.
Bl17	Stimulates Blood circulation, strengthens weakness in whole body, disperses fullness in diaphragm.
Bl18	Eliminates Damp-Heat and stagnation of Qi, calms Liv and GB.
Bl19	Eliminates Heat from Liv and GB, calms St Qi.
Bl20	Regulates function of Sp and eliminates Damp, strengthens Blood.
Bl21	Dispels Damp and removes stagnation, regulates St Qi.
Bl22	Regulates movement of water in Lower Heater.
Bl23	Eliminates Damp, regulates Ki Qi.
Bl24	Strengthens Qi, 'Shu point of lumbar area'.
Bl25	Stimulates function of LI.
Bl26	'Shu point of sacral area'.
Bl28	Disperses Qi of Lower Heater, regulates Bl function.
Bl29	Exit Barrier point.

Bl32	Stimulates Ki Qi and regulates Lower Heater; helps relieve stagnation of blood in uterus.
Bl43	Warms Lu and makes Qi go down.
Bl54	Stimulates the meridians and removes obstruction from them.
Bl37	Regulates circulation of Blood and Qi in meridians in waist and legs.
Bl38	Regulates transformation of water in Lower Heater.
Bl40	Dispels Damp, removes Heat from Blood.
Bl60	Eliminates internal Wind, general pain, chronic lumbago.
Bl62	Stimulates the meridians, key point of Yang Chiao.
Bl63	Entry Barrier point.
Bl64	Dispels Internal Wind.
Bl67	Much used in childbirth, can move position of foetus.
Ki1	Stimulates Ki Yin, calms the Fire of Ht.
Ki2	Calms Fire and cools the Blood (combine with Liv3).
Ki3	Tonifies Ki Qi, calms the Fire.
Ki5	Entry and exit Barrier point.
Ki6	Makes Ki Yin ascend to throat (use with Lu7), eliminates Heat.
Ki7	Nourishes Ki Yin, eliminates Damp-Heat.
Ki9	Stimulates Ki Yin, stimulates Yin Wei Mai.
Ki10	Tonifies Ki, dispels Heat, regulates Lower Heater.
Pe2	Entry Barrier point.
Pe3	Frees Ht Qi, dispels Heat from Blood.
Pe4	Exit Barrier point, calms the Ht.
Pe5	Removes internal Heat and Phlegm from Ht.
Pe6	Moves stagnation in Middle Heater, regulates circulation of Qi, calms Ht and mind.
Pe7	Disperses Fire of Ht, calms Ht, mind and St.
Pe8	Disperses Fire of Ht.
Pe9	Disperses Fire of Ht.
TH3	Regulates Qi, disperses pathogenic Heat.
TH4	Stimulates the Three Heaters, relaxes the tendons.
TH5	Dispels Wind, relaxes tendons, removes blockage in Yang Wei Mai and so helps exterior symptoms.
TH6	Removes stagnation, particularly in the bowels, generally helps the Qi circulation, balances the function of the Three Heaters.
TH7	Entry Barrier point.
TH13	Exit Barrier point.
TH17	Disperses Internal Wind.
TH23	Dispels Wind and clears Fire.

GB1	Clears Wind-Heat, dispels Fire.
GB2	Eliminates Wind and clears the meridians.
GB12	Eliminates Wind.
GB14	Clears Internal Wind.
GB20	Eliminates Internal Wind, calms the Yang, calms the Liv.
GB24	Eliminates Damp-Heat.
GB30	Moves obstruction in the meridians.
GB31	Dispels Wind, relaxes tendons.
GB33	Exit Barrier point.
GB34	Removes Damp-Heat, removes Phlegm-Fire in St, calms Li Yang, tonifies tendons (combine with TH6 for 'Wandering Bi').
GB36	Entry Barrier point.
GB39	Dispels Wind and Damp, tonifies Bone Marrow.
GB40	Stimulates Liv and GB, invigorates the meridians.
GB41	Dispels Damp-Heat, holds down Liv Qi, key point of Dai Mai.
Liv2	Eliminates Liv Fire, moves stagnation of Qi, clears Lower Heater.
Liv3	Regulates circulation of Qi and Blood, calms Liv and GB.
Liv5	Eliminates Damp-Heat from genital area.
Liv6	Exit Barrier point.
Liv8	Dispels Damp-Heat, nourishes Liv Yin, clears Lower Heater, relaxes tendons.
Liv11	Entry Barrier point.
Liv13	Moves stagnation in St and helps in transformation in Sp, regulates circulation of Qi and Blood and helps Liv function.
Liv14	Regulates circulation of Qi and Blood, helps function of Liv and GB.
GV1	Regulates balance between Du Mai and Ren Mai and removes blockages in them.
GV3	Makes Yang go out and down, eliminates Cold-Damp and regulates Ki Qi.
GV4	Strengthens Ki Qi and tonifies the Yang.
GV9	Regulates circulation of Qi and removes fullness in chest and diaphragm, soothes Liv and GB.
GV14	Governs all the Yang channels, makes the Yang go out and up, eliminates Wind-Cold.
GV16	Lower meeting point for marrow, eliminates internal Wind.
GV20	Summons energy to the head, eliminates Wind.
GV23	Eliminates Wind-Heat, particularly in the nasal area.
GV26	Revival point, eliminates Wind.

CV3	Regulates Lower Heater and eliminates Damp-Heat, regulates and strengthens the function of the uterus.
CV4	Makes the Yin go out and down, tonifies the Blood and the Yuan Qi, regulates the menses.
CV6	Regulates Qi circulation and dispels Damp, tonifies weakness.
CV12	Stimulates St and Sp and transforms Mucus, calms ascending Qi of St.
CV14	Moves the Ht Qi, calms the St.
CV17	Stimulates Lu Qi and transforms Mucus, regulates the Qi circulation and subdues ascending Qi of St.
CV22	Makes the Yin go out and up, subdues ascending Qi and regulates Qi circulation, helps dispersing function of Lu (CV22 and St 40 combined make mucus descend).
CV24	Dispels Wind.

Examples

Dysmenorrhoea

Pain in this condition is usually because things are not moving.

One possible cause is Stagnant Qi, which fails to move the blood giving rise to pain either before or during the menses. Use GB41 (to loosen Dai Mai), CV6 (to move the Qi), Liv2, Sp8 (for congealed blood and also to affect the uterus) and CV3 (affects the uterus). Can add tonification of CV4 to tonify the original Qi.

Another cause is Congealed Blood. This is usually a much more painful condition, with clots, and the patient feels better once these have been passed. The Blood tends to be dark and purplish, and the pulse is choppy. Tonify LI4 and disperse Sp6, Sp8, Sp10, St25 and St29.

Stomach ache

This can arise from cold and emptiness, with a cold clear discharge and a spasmodic type of pain, loose inoffensive stools and clear urine. One needs to warm St and Sp via Sp2, St36, Bl20 and CV12.

Another cause is excess Heat in St and Sp. The patient is usually constipated and thirsty, and has dark, concentrated urine and foul-smelling stools. One could use points such as St43 (to cool St), St45 and St37.

Vertigo

This is frequently a symptom of Liv Fire blazing upwards, with the usual red face, irritability, hyperactivity, bitter taste in mouth, possible tinnitus, etc. Calm Liv2, GB20, GB38, Bl18, Bl19, Bl47 and Bl48.

5

Other considerations

So far we have dealt with the 'rules' of acupuncture, but there are other aspects of point selection which, whilst not strictly rules, have to be borne in mind if we are to formulate the best possible prescription, and amongst the foremost of these is the use of reunion points and a consideration of the internal pathways. These latter are not only the means by which the external meridians communicate with their appropriate organ, but they are also the means by which the various meridians are linked to each other – sometimes via the principal meridians, sometimes via the tendino-muscular or the divergent meridians.

Special points, such as GV14 and GV20, are meeting places of all the Yang meridians, but several other points are also of great importance, such as St12 (Quepen), which is the meeting place of the principal meridians of LI, TH, GB, SI and the tendino-muscular meridian of the Lu, and Bl1 (Jingming), the meeting point of St, SI, TH, Bl, the divergent meridians of St, Sp, SI, Ht, the Yang Chiao and the Yin Chiao.

As a point of interest, we might take the true path of the Gall Bladder meridian, which runs not from GB29 to GB30, but from GB29 to Bl31 and Bl33 and then to GB30. This accounts for the point GB30 proving effective in cases of pain in the posterior branch of the sciatic nerve (the course of the Bl meridian). There is also a linkage between St30 (Qichong) and the GB meridian, accounting for the use of St30 in cases of arthritic hip (apart from its local use). One can augment this with the use of the *opposite* action on St5 (Daying), which is also connected to the GB line.

One can also cite SI12 (Bingfeng), the meeting place of SI, LI, TH and GB – which is why affections of the Shao Tai Yang (SI) at the trapezius can sometimes radiate into the arm down the LI line rather than down that of the SI line itself. In such cases SI12 is the obvious point to use.

Table 5.1 shows where each meridian unites, and which meridian each point connects with.

Table 5.1

Meridian	Unites with:	Connects with:
Lu	St at St12 via T/Ms LI at LI18 via D/Ms Pe and Ht via T/Ms at GB22 Sp at Lu1	Lu1 – Sp
LI	St at LI20, St12, St25, St37, CV24, GV26; T/M at St3 SI at SI12; SI T/M at GB13 GB at SI12, GB3–6, GB14; Longitudinal Luo at St12 TH at TH20; TH T/M at GB13 Lu at LI18 (D/M) and LI1 (internal branch) CV at CV3, CV24 GV at GV14, GV26 Yang Chiao at LI15, 16	LI15 – Yang Chiao LI16 – Yang Chiao LI18 – D/Ms of Lu LI 20–St
St	LI at St12, St25, St37, CV24, GV26 Sp at St40, St42 SI at SI1, St39, St12 BI at St1, GV24 TH at St12 GB at St5, St12, St30 Chong Mai at St30 Yang Chiao at St1–3 Yang Wei at St8	St1 – BI, Yang Chiao St3 – Yang Chiao St4 – LI, Yang Chiao St5 – GB St6 – GB St8 – GB, Yang Wei St12 – LI, TH, GB, SI, T/M of Lu St25 – LI St30 – GB St37 – LI St39 – SI St40 – Sp St42 – Sp
Sp	Lu at Lu1 Ht at CV17, HT1 Ki at Sp6, Sp13 Liv at Sp6, Sp12, Sp13, Liv14 GB at GB24 Yin Wei at Sp13, Sp15, Sp16	Sp6 – Liv, Ki Sp12 – Liv Sp13 – Liv, Ki, Yin Wei Sp15 – Yin Wei Sp16 – Yin Wei
Ht	BI1 via D/M Sp at Ht1 Lu and Pe via T/Ms at GB22	Ht1 – Sp
SI	LI at SI12, St12 St at St12, CV12, BI1 BI at BI1, BI11, BI36, CV12 TH at TH20, TH22, SI12, SI19, St12, CV12, CV17 GB at SI12, SI19, St12, GB7–12 Lu at St12, CV12 Sp at CV17	SI10 – Yang Chiao, Yang Wei SI12 – LI, TH, GB SI15 – GV SI18 – TH, GB SI19 – TH, GB

Table 5.1 Continued

Meridian	Unites with:	Connects with:
	Ht at CV17 Liv at CV17 Yang Wei at SI10 Yang Chiao at SI10	
Bl	St at GV24 Si at Bl1, Bl11, Bl36, GV13 Th at GV13, Bl53 GB at GB8–12, Bl31, Bl33, GB30 Liv at Bl33 Yang Chiao at Bl1, Bl59, Bl61, Bl62 Yin Chiao at Bl1 Yang Wei at Bl63	Bl – St, SI, TH (also D/Ms of St, Sp, SI, Ht, Yang Chiao, Yin Chiao) Bl11 – SI, GB, Lu Bl31 – GB Bl32 – GB Bl33 – GB, Liv Bl41 – SI Bl43 – SI Bl39 – TH (visceral aspect) Bl59 – Yang Chiao Bl61 – Yang Chiao Bl62 – Yang Chiao Bl63 – Yang Wei
Ki	Sp at Sp6, CV3, CV4 Liv at Sp6, CV3, CV4, Ki25 Pe at Ki25, CV17 GV at GV1 CV at CV3, CV4, CV17 Yin Chiao at Ki2, Ki6, Ki8 Yin Wei at Ki9 Chong Mai at Ki11–21	Ki6 – Yin Chiao Ki8 – Yin Chiao Ki9 – Yin Wei Ki25 – Pe, Liv
Pe	Ht at CV17 Liv at Pe1 GB at Pe1 TH at CV17 (Upper Heater at CV17, Middle Heater at CV12, Lower Heater at CV7)	Pe1 – GB, Liv
TH	LI at SI12, St12, TH20 St at St12, GB4, GB5, GB14, Bl1 SI at SI12, SI18, SI19, TH22 Bl at Bl1 GB at SI12, GB21, St12, GB1, GB4, GB5, TH17, TH20, TH22 Pe at CV17 GV at GV14 Yang Wei at TH5, TH13, TH15	TH15 – GB, Yang Chiao TH16 – GB Th17 – GB TH20 – LI, SI, GB TH21 – Si, GB TH22 – SI, GB
GB	Lu at Bl11, St12 LI at SI12, St12, GB3, GB14 St at St12, GB3, GB4, GB5, GB14, GB21, GB30, St5, St6 Sp at GB24	GB1 – SI, TH GB3 – LI, St, TH GB4 – LI, St, TH GB5 – LI, St, TH GB6 – LI

Table 5.1 Continued

Meridian	Unites with:	Connects with:
	SI at BI11, SI12, SI18, SI19, GB1, GB7–10, GB12, GB15	GB7 – BI, SI, TH
	BI at BI11, BI31, BI33, GB7–12	GB8 – BI, SI
	GB14, GB15, GB30	GB9 – BI, SI
	TH at TH16, SI12, St12, GB1	GB10 – BI, SI
	GB3–5, GB7, GB11, GB14, GB15, GB20, GB21	GB11 – BI
	Yang Chiao at GB20, GB29	GB12 – BI, SI
	Yang Wei at GB13–20, GB21	GB13 – Yang Wei
	GB35	GB14 – LI, St, BI, TH, Yang Wei
	Dai Mai at GB26–28	GB15 – BI, SI, TH, Yang Wei
		GB16 – Yang Wei
		GB17 – Yang Wei
		GB18 – Yang Wei
		GB19 – Yang Wei
		GB20 – TH
		GB21 – St, TH
		GB22 – T/Ms of Lu, Ht, Pe
		GB24 – Sp
		GB26 – Dai Mai
		GB27 – Dai Mai
		GB28 – Dai Mai
		GB29 – Yang Chiao
		GB30 – BI
		GB35 – Yang Wei
Liv	Sp at Sp6, Sp12, Sp13, Liv14	Liv14 – Sp, GB
	GB at Liv14	
	Ki at Sp6	
	CV at CV2–4	
	GV at GV20	
	Yin Wei at Liv14	
CV		CV2 – Liv
		CV3 – LI, Sp, Ki, Liv
		CV4 – Sp, Ki, Liv
		CV7 – Ht, Pe
		CV9 – Lu
		CV12 – Lu, Pe (central point of five Yang organs)
		CV17 – SI, TH, Lu, Ht, Pe, Ki, Liv
		CV22 – Yin Wei
		CV23 – Yin Wei
		CV24 – LI
GV		GV1 – Ki
		GV13 – BI, TH
		GV14 – Central point of all Yang meridians
		GV15 – BI, Yang Wei
		GV16 – BI, Yang Wei
		GV20 – Central reunion point
		GV24 – St, BI
		GV26 – LI

6

Needle techniques

Once we have taken all the foregoing into consideration and have decided upon the points we think will best serve our purpose, the next obvious step is to decide which points need stimulating and which need sedating, and how best to achieve this.

The whole business of 'toning' and 'draining' has been vastly over-complicated by some of the teaching emanating from mainland China, especially the statement that 'reducing is strong stimulation'.

To start from the beginning, if a condition has too much energy it needs reducing, sedating, calming, draining – call it what you will, there is too much there, so we have to reduce it. If there is a lack of energy or some attribute we have to add to it (or tonify or stimulate) and to do this, in theory, we either add the missing or weak attribute (which could be Heat, Cold, Dryness, Qi or whatever) or bring it from somewhere else in the body.

Complications set in when we start to consider the basic cause of the imbalance – and that word 'imbalance' is the clue to the whole treatment. Fundamental to Chinese thought is that matter and energy are interchangeable, and that matter is simply condensed energy. The energy flows through its well-defined pathways – the meridians, both internal and external – in an orderly progression (see Low, 1983) and reaches its maximum at various parts of its pathway at various times (refer to both the concept of the Chinese Clock and the Celestial Stems). Any interference with this energy flow causes a blockage – a 'stuckness' in the energy – which will produce an over-abundance in one part with a concomitant deficiency in another. We are therefore faced with the task of either:

1 removing the blockage – and this in itself may restore the correct flow and function with no further treatment being required, or
2 transferring energy from where there is too much to where there is too little.

I have repeatedly used the word 'energy' because this is the most convenient to use. In this context we have to remember that energy is derived from nourishment and nourishment is carried by the blood.

It is therefore stated that 'the blood supplies the Qi and the Qi drives the blood' – which is self-evident if one cares to think about it. As an added complication the Qi energy is considered to work in several different ways, which means it manifests its activity in several different functions, and each functional energy is given a different name. Hence we have Jung Qi, Ching Qi, Wei Qi, etc., not to mention Ku Qi and Ta Qi, and each of the aspects of Qi can be affected by the choice of point.

It is also considered by some that the amount of energy in the body is a constant, but I would disagree most strongly indeed with this statement. The 'ancestral' energy – our basic inherited substratum – is naturally fixed from the moment of conception, but our other energies – our post-heaven blood and Qi – will be subject to the innumerable influences of food, mood, climate and season, all of which will affect the way in which a patient will react and respond to treatment. Whether it is possible to actually 'put energy into a patient' is a very moot point. Advice on lifestyle – feeding, resting, exercise – will all improve the basic energy on all levels, and it can also be affected by the exhibition of the appropriate herbal medicines, but the idea that one can introduce energy with a needle is rather naïve. There is a statement that 'needles transfer the energy, moxa puts energy in', and although I rather like the idea that moxa actually introduces energy, I don't really believe it. What moxa does is increase the local circulation and this increased blood flow will bring nourishment (and therefore energy) to the area. It will also have its natural corollaries of warming and drying and, importantly, the rubefacient action will 'flush away' impurities and blockages and allow the energy to flow smoothly. It has also been shown that stimulation by needle can increase the local circulation, whilst it is possible that there will be a local as well as a general increase in the endorphin level.

With regard to the statement about reducing being strong stimulation, in the British Acupuncture College I am repeatedly citing the example that every action, taken past a certain level, causes an equal and opposite reaction, and a good illustration of this is a cold bath – jump into it and at first it stimulates, but stay in it for a long period and it becomes enervating. The ultimate example is acupuncture analgesia, where the stimulation is carried to such a length that the pertained meridian and/or organ is rendered incapable of producing the sensation of pain. Even moxa can have a similar effect – too strong an application can burn, but too long can render the point incapable of further reaction.

The very simplest application is where to stimulate; one inserts a needle, manipulates it to summon the energy (obtain Dai Qi) and then removes it as soon as the energy arrives. To sedate; one inserts the needle, stimulates it to obtain Dai Qi and then leaves it alone for about 20 minutes before removal. This effect can be enhanced by tying it in with the patient's breathing, as shown in Table 6.1.

Table 6.1 Basic needle technique

	Sedate	Supply
Insertion	Fast	Slow
During	Inspiration	Expiration
Then	Summon energy and leave about 20 minutes	Summon energy and withdraw after a few seconds
Withdrawal	Slow	Fast
During	Expiration	Inspiration
Then	Leave	Close hole by rubbing

One can augment the 'balancing' effect (depending upon the patient's strength and build) by restimulating the energy every few minutes to keep the Qi moving. This is called the Even Method. I have actually heard it said that one applies this method if one is not sure whether to sedate or to stimulate, but this is a rather naïve approach and to my mind demonstrates an inability to grasp any type of feeling for what is happening in the area of the point once the needle is inserted. The stimulation is by the well-known 'twisting and thrusting' technique, and the flow of Qi can be directed by slanting the needle in the direction in which one wishes the Qi to flow. In theory one can increase the supplying action by slanting the needle in the direction of the flow of energy in the meridian and sedate by opposing or going against it. Whether there is any difference obtainable by clockwise or anticlockwise rotation is problematical – the various references are conflicting, but in any case there will be a slight variation in rotational bias due to practitioners being right- or left-handed.

A further interesting method for increasing the flow of Qi is the so-called 'pressing needling'. The practitioner inserts the needle in the direction in which he wishes the Qi to flow, and maintaining his hold on the handle with one hand whilst keeping up a strong clockwise bias he percusses up the length of the meridian with the other hand.

Of great important is the angle of needle insertion. Needles may be inserted vertically (at right angles to the skin), obliquely (at 45° to the skin), or horizontally (almost flat along the skin). For the latter, nip the skin up into a fold before inserting. This technique is used for the majority of points where there is no depth of underlying tissue, also where specific indications exist. All points other than those following are usually used with a vertical insertion:

Lu7	To affect thumb, slope to thumb
	To affect meridian, slope to Lu8
Lu11	Oblique
LI1	Oblique to LI2
LI4	Direct towards Pe8
LI15	Oblique downwards
LI20	Horizontally to Bl1
St2	Downwards to St3
St4	Towards St6
St5	Towards St6
St6	Towards St4, or vertically
St8	Towards TH23
St35	Into joint, towards Liv8
Sp1	Oblique to Sp2
Sp17–21	Oblique, 1 cm
Ht7	Usually towards Ht8
Ht9	Oblique
SI1	Oblique
SI18	Towards St4, or vertically
SI19	Vertically, with mouth open
Bl2	Horizontally to Bl3 or laterally
Bl3–8	Horizontally upwards
Bl9	Horizontally downwards
Bl12	Oblique to Bl41
Bl60	To tip of medial malleolus
Bl67	Oblique
Ki3	To tip of lateral malleolus
Pe1	Oblique
Pe9	Oblique
TH1	Oblique
TH2	Towards TH4
TH20	Oblique downwards
TH22	Oblique downwards
TH23	Horizontally posteriorly
GB1	Horizontally posteriorly/laterally
GB4–11	Horizontally posteriorly

GB12	Horizontally downwards
GB13	Horizontally upwards
GB14	Horizontally downwards
GB15	Horizontally upwards
GB16–19	Horizontally posteriorly
GB20	Towards tip of nose (or horizontally to GV16 for torticollis)
GB40	Towards Ki3
GB43	Oblique upwards
GB44	Oblique
Liv1	Oblique
Liv2	Oblique to underneath hallux
Liv5	Horizontally
Liv6	Horizontally
GV2	Oblique upwards
GV9	Oblique upwards
GV12	Vertical or oblique to right or left as symptoms require (even two crossed if symptoms bilateral)
GV17–24	Horizontally under skin
GV26	Oblique upwards
GV28	Oblique upwards
CV15	Oblique downwards
CV16–21	Horizontally under skin
CV22	Oblique posteriorly/inferiorly
CV24	Oblique upwards

The one factor all agree to be of paramount importance is the obtaining of deqi (or Dai Qi). This is usually described as feeling like a numb, spreading ache, hopefully travelling along the course of the meridian towards the affected organ or area, but this is subject to individual variations. Patients will vary in their sensitivity and this in itself will act as a sort of regulator – an area which is hypersensitive does not call for much stimulation, whilst one which is hypoactive will obviously require considerably more to produce the necessary reaction. The patient's own pain threshold will serve to keep the practitioner informed about this!

We have said that the normal sensation is a numbish distended feeling. The patient should be asked to differentiate between a feeling of pain and a strong sensation. Once they have grasped the idea that there is a definite distinction they will be able to cooperate much more fully, as deqi should *not* be acutely painful. A sudden acute pain like an electric shock running down a limb is usually a sign that the practitioner has hit a nerve by mistake, although some Chinese writers regard this as a good sign in certain chronic disorders such as sciatica, hemiplegia, etc. However, it must be borne in mind that some points are definitely painful 'in their own right', particularly the Tsing or End Points, most points on the sole of the foot and GV26 (Renzhong), and I always warn the patient about this likelihood. An interesting reaction is when the patient describes a sensation of 'water travelling down under the skin' whilst the needle is static in the point. This is obviously due to the Qi energy moving on its own, and will usually precede an excellent result.

I have mentioned the importance of needle angles. Needle depth is of equal import, because an impulsive practitioner can easily thrust a needle too deeply and actually go *through* the point. The patient will feel no deqi, but on lifting the needle back to the correct depth deqi is immediate – this factor can lead to interesting speculation as to the actual physical and material structure of the meridians.

Very superficial needling will produce a different sensation entirely, with a tingling feeling spreading around the needle surrounded by a red patch of about 2.5 cm diameter. Whether one calls it 'the evil Yang coming out' or whether one refers to an 'epicritic reaction', it is obviously a reaction of the Wei energy and can produce very strong results on this level. This visible redness around the needle appears in the majority of cases where there is a Wei energy involvement and is manifestly due to capillary dilatation.

Where there is a lot of heat around, the use of judicious blood-letting is often advocated, calling for the extraction of a few drops of blood from the point. Traditionally this is achieved by the use of a special prismatic or triangular needle, but personally I find that the use of a spring-loaded lancet is more effective. What has to be kept in mind in this approach is that the ratio of blood to energy in the meridians varies from one meridian to another (see Low, 1983), and whilst the Tai Yang (Bl and SI) has more blood than energy and bleeding is therefore frequently highly desirable, the Shao Yin (Ki and Ht) has more energy than blood, and bleeding on either of these lines should definitely be avoided.

We have already described the basic, simple approach to 'reducing' and tonification, but there are of course many more advanced and more sophisticated needle manipulations designed for more specific effects. These are all based upon eight standard rules:

1 Liu Chen (Wo Chen) – Resting Needle: leave needle inserted for 20 minutes in sedation.
2 Ts'o – To Rotate: when needle has reached proper depth.
3 Nien – To Rotate: during insertion or withdrawal.
4 Yao – To Rock the Needle.

5 Fei – To Shake the Needle: up and down, quick trembling.
6 P'an – To Transfer: this rule requires the needle to be inserted into different directions from the same superficial point.
7 An – To Arrange: requires the needle to be inserted into three levels – superficial, medium and deep.
8 Shen – To Spread: the needle is withdrawn in three levels, from deep to medium to superficial.

These elementary manipulations are combined into many precise techniques.

Superficial points

When we insert into a superficial point we must know upon which energy we wish to act, either Wei or Jung.

Example

LI2 is indicated in local joint troubles and also as a specific point for constipation. In the first, local case, we must act on the superficial Wei energy. In the second, organic disorder, we must act on the deep Jung energy.

Supply

1 Wei energy (Wo Ma Yao Ling) 'The Hungry Horse Shakes his Bell'. After the needle is in, rotate the handle slowly at an extreme angle to one side and at a smaller angle to the other. Such action, whilst ineffective on the Jung energy where the point of the needle is, is maximum at the level of the skin, that of the Wei energy, and the skin clings almost immediately. Supply is thus to the Wei energy (Fig. 6.1).

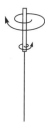

Figure 6.1

2 Jung energy (Ch'ing Long Pai Wei) 'The Dragon Moves his Tail'.
Here the movement of the needle must be ineffective superficially but
strongest deep at the point of the needle. The name shows how the
needle is to move (Fig. 6.2).

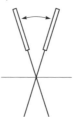

Figure 6.2

3 After insertion, manipulate the needle as if it were the rudder of a
boat, very slowly and longitudinally (along line). The needle is a
lever of the first order, with the skin surface the fulcrum of
movement, and therefore the Wei energy is not affected (fulcrum
motionless), but the point of the needle performs scraping in the
depth, effective in supplying Jung energy.

These rules obey the principle of supplying being quick intervention,
therefore manipulate during three to seven complete breaths of the
patient.

Sedate

1 Wei energy (Pai Hu Yao T'ou) 'The White Tiger Shakes his Head'.
This is comparable to the previous rule of the rudder of a boat, but
this is quite opposite, with drainage of the Wei whilst the previous
one supplies Jung. The movement is also lateral, but as a lever of the
second order, and the fulcrum is now the point of the needle, with no
influence at the point where lies the Jung energy. Most effect is at the
level of the skin and the Wei energy – it enlarges the needle hole
without hurting the Jung energy (Fig. 6.3).

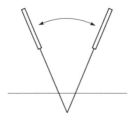

Figure 6.3

2 Jung energy (Fong Huan Shau Ch'ih) 'The Male and Female Phoenix Ruffle their Wings'. After the needle is in, apply rotation to the handle, but a periodic one, in both directions equally: rotate, stop, rotate, stop, etc. As we are in the field of sedation, during pauses we must leave the handle, but must also rotate quickly, with a very small angle in both directions. The point of the needle has a noticeable movement in the depth (opposite to law Supply 1), but the angle is small and so avoids touching the Wei of the skin.

These two drainage rules take a long time of action – at least 10–15 minutes.

Deep points (two levels)

Into deep or medium-depth points the previous rules are possible, but we have to consider a new tissue – the muscles. In all muscular symptoms, whether excess or deficiency, it is best to apply the two following rules. Since the trouble is deep, we must find the normal energy as a reference, and here we use the superficial Wei (Fig. 6.4).

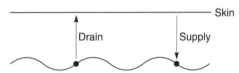

Figure 6.4

Supply

In the case of symptoms of deficiency of deep energy the points are needled by the rule Long Hu Sheng Chiang ('The Dragon and the Tiger go Up and Down'). The purpose is to supply, i.e. drive normal superficial energy to the depth where the energy is deficient.

Insert the needle very slowly into the skin only, then rotate quickly in both directions at the same angle to summon the Wei. When it arrives (skin clings) transfer to the depth by driving the needle to the proper depth slowly, without rotating, then withdraw at once quickly, with a strong rotation at the same angle in both directions (Fig. 6.5).

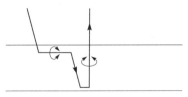

Figure 6.5

When the needle is out, since we are supplying do not forget to rub the hole to close it.

Symbolically, the Dragon is the superficial Yang energy going to the depth to divert or dispel the deep excess of Yin, the Tiger.

Sedate

With excess in depth we must bring it to the surface to disperse it. The rule is Tzü Wu Tao Chin ('To Strike the Hours from Midnight to Midday').

Insert the needle according to the drainage rule – quickly with rotation, but on a bias towards 12 o'clock directly to the depth. Then wait a few moments and withdraw slowly without rotation but only to the skin level, then insert again towards 1 o'clock (with the drainage rule). Wait a few moments, withdraw and repeat towards 2 o'clock. Carry on round towards 12 o'clock. To apply the rule of duration, time with the patient's breathing as shown in Fig. 6.6.

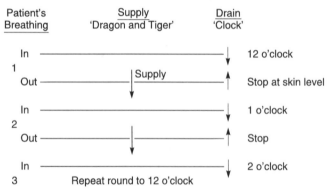

Figure 6.6

Acupuncture at three levels – deep and medium-depth points

We sometimes have to act at three levels – superficial, deep and medium.

Superficial	– T'ien P'ing	– Heaven
Medium depth	– Jen P'ing	– Man
Deep	– Ti P'ing	– Earth

When acting successively on each of the three, try to harmonize superficial Wei, deep Jung and their synthesis Jen P'ing (half Wei, half

Jung). Such an energic manipulation is indicated into all deep or medium-depth command points, i.e. points of the Five Elements, Yuan points, Luo points, Key points of the Irregular vessels, and all Back Shu points. The paramedian Bladder line is somatic, on the sympathetic ganglia. The external branch is the psychic control, 'the spirit of the organ', i.e. Bl52 commands the Will.

Supply

Shao Shan Huo ('The Fire of the Volcano'). Insert slowly, with no rotation, during expiration. Stop at the superficial level and rotate until the next expiration. Energy comes and the skin clings. During the second expiration drive slowly to medium depth with tremble. Stop at medium depth and again rotate. On next expiration drive slowly with tremble to the depth, on inspiration withdraw quickly with rotation to medium level. Wait until next inspiration and withdraw quickly with rotation. Rub hole to close it (Fig. 6.7).

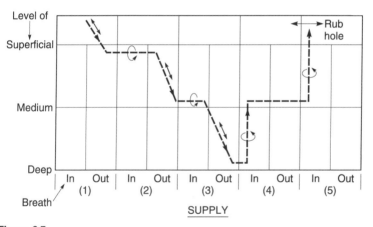

Figure 6.7

Drainage

T'u T'ien Liang ('The Penetration of Celestial Freshness'). Insert quickly with rotation, directly to the depth, during first inspiration. Leave, and wait until second expiration when withdraw slowly with tremble to the medium depth. Wait until next expiration when withdraw slowly with tremble to the superficial level. On inspiration insert quickly with rotation to the depth, leave until second expiration when withdraw completely, slowly with tremble. Leave the hole (Fig. 6.8).

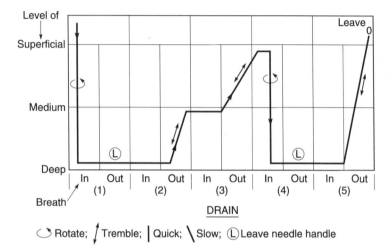

Figure 6.8

In spite of the same duration of action we can notice that the general principles are respected in that drainage is longer than supplying – there is one breath difference.

Double action

Remember the case for opposite action – drain the remote point whilst local points are supplied, etc. Actually, the opposite action on remote points gives quite good results, but for complete success a double action is preferable.

Example: lumbar pain

This is treated by local drainage to Bl23, supply Bl40, but this is even better when the supplying action is completed by a drainage one, i.e. when a point is indicated with opposite action it is always best to complete with the same action as on the local one.

● Drain Bl23 (local).
● Supply Bl40 (remote).
● Drain Bl40, without withdrawing the needle.
● To treat Bl40 insert supplying needle, withdraw to skin and manipulate as in Fig. 6.9.

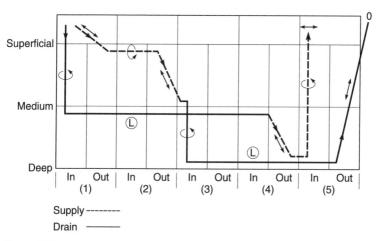

Figure 6.9

- The converse can also apply:
  Supply → Drain
  Drain → Supply
- This is known as Long Hu Chiao Chan ('The Battle of the Tiger and the Dragon').

7

Moxa techniques

The use of needles is, of course, only one of numerous techniques utilized by Chinese medicine. The term 'acupuncture' is, by its very name, actually limited to the use of needles alone – the Chinese name is 'Chen-Chiu', which means 'needle-moxa' – and in practice the two modalities are indivisible and complementary.

At the start of the previous chapter we discussed the concept of moxa actually 'putting energy in'. Mukoto Yamashita, in his book *Introductory Text of Acupuncture for Meridian Therapy* (1971), states:

> There are three meanings to tonification in practice. The first is the general meaning of drawing and collecting Qi to increase its amount. The second is to gently loosen Qi and Blood which has become stagnant to allow it to flow away so that fresh normal Qi can be drawn in. The circulation of fresh Qi and Blood is thereby encouraged. The third meaning is to add Qi. The first and second types of tonification are used when a patient has ample physical strength, but the third type is necessary in cases of severe debilitation when Qi must be added from the outside. In these cases, warming tonification by moxibustion is the most effective method.

For a more detailed study of moxibustion generally, the reader is referred to *The Principles and Practice of Moxibustion* (Newman Turner and Low, 1981), but the major considerations are:

1 Basically, moxa warms and moves the Qi and Blood, which means it gets things moving and relieves stagnation. It generally dispels cold, tends to disperse toxins (because of the anti-toxic nature of fresh blood brought to the area), and strengthens Ki Yang.
2 There are two traditional forms of application – direct and indirect – with direct implying the application of moxa directly into contact with the skin surface, and indirect with the heat being applied either to some other substance placed on the skin, or by the use of a moxa roll or Akabane stick.
3 The use of heated needles, which direct the heat more precisely into the point and will also cause it to travel more into the meridian rather than in an area.

To consider first of all direct moxibustion, this invariably implies the use of cones of moxa punk, which are used in three different sizes – large (about 1 cm in diameter), medium (about the size of an olive stone), and small (the size of a grain of wheat). The Japanese frequently use very small cones, the size of grains of rice.

One uses the large cones on thickly muscled areas such as the shoulders, low back and buttocks, the medium cones on the abdomen and limbs, and the smallest ones where the skin is thin, such as the hands, feet and back of the neck. The number used follows roughly the same rules, although traditionally one uses, for a female, the patient's age divided by seven and, for a male, the age divided by eight. This implies that the greater the age the less the reaction produced and hence the greater the stimulus required, but this approach has to be tempered by consideration of:

● an elderly patient not being able to take too much stimulation;
● possible weakness in skin tone and circulation.

Some points are actually specified as requiring one moxa for every year of the patient's age to a maximum of 40. These would naturally call for the smallest cones. Empty and cold conditions are the ones which would call for the greater number of large cones.

Direct moxa itself was traditionally used in three forms:

1 Non-scarring – used for empty and cold diseases.
2 Blistering (with small cones) – used mainly in asthma and tuberculosis.
3 Scarring – where the cone burnt right down to the skin. For rather obvious reasons this method is now obsolete, even though one of the classics advises that, for maximum effect, the Sanli point (St36) should be kept moist, i.e. in a perpetual state of semi-suppuration!

The first form of indirect moxa is where the cone is placed on top of a slice of some other substance. In theory, the effect of the moxa is enhanced by the absorption of medicinal substances from the slice into the point and the two most common substances used are ginger or garlic. To quote from Newman Turner and Low (1981):

> On Ginger (Gejiang juifa). A slice of ginger 1 to 3 fen (a fen is a tenth of a cun or 'acupuncture inch', which will vary according to its location or the patient's build, see Chapter 11) thick, with tiny holes pierced in it, is placed under the cone. If the pain is too violent remove until it subsides, then replace the cone and ginger and keep it there until the patient perspires and the point becomes red. There is danger of blistering if the heat is not regulated.

> On garlic (Gesuan juifa). Used as above, but when the pain is felt it should not be removed. Used for chronic paralysis or for the early

stages of a carbuncle, and on the spot where it dries out from the underlying inflammation one places a slice of garlic about 3 fen thick with the moxa cone on top. Change the garlic after five cones. If the carbuncle is painful, cauterise until the pain disappears; if not painful, cauterise until it becomes so. If no suppuration occurs one can apply long-lasting cauterisation. If the carbuncle has several heads, spread squashed garlic over it before applying the cone.

Other substances are also recommended in the literature, but the above two are easily the most commonly used. The others include moxa on chives, aconite, white pepper, fermented soya beans, fine clay, onion and shallot.

One special application is for the use of moxa on CV8, the navel, where the specific technique calls for the navel to be filled with sea salt and the moxa cone burnt on top of the salt. It is used mainly for acute gastroenteritis, chronic intestinal diseases and diarrhoea, although it is also useful in cases of general debility due to empty Ki Yang, when one adds chives and musk to the salt, then burns a 1 cm chunk of moxa (cut from a roll) on a slice of ginger.

As with the standard concept of strong stimulation producing a reducing effect, one can 'reduce' with moxa by fanning or blowing on the cone to make it burn more quickly and fiercely. This technique is particularly applicable to pain over the acromial process, where the rule calls for three large 'blown' moxas right on the spot (see Low, 1987 p. 38).

The commonest usage of indirect moxa is the moxa roll. I use the ordinary 'mild' moxa roll (which is pure artemesia) mainly for children and elderly patients and also for chopping up into chunks to burn on the needle (see later). The medicated rolls, such as the Tai I and Nien Ying, have other substances added to the artemesia to make them burn hotter and are thus better for use in Wind, Cold and Damp Bi, flaccid paralysis and Empty-Cold syndromes. One uses either a 'spreading' or 'pecking' technique, depending upon the effect desired, whilst for use on a very small area, such as over the end of Tsing points, an Akabane or Japanese greenstick may be found to be preferable to a roll.

The main difference between direct and indirect is that with direct moxa the action is immediate and the effect longer lasting, whilst with the indirect (especially with the roll) it is slower to take effect and its results are of a shorter duration. My own feelings are that the difference is similar to that found between radiant heat and infrared – the direct penetrates more deeply, the indirect effect is more on the surface.

The basic rules are:

1 If points on the legs and arms are to be used, moxa the arms first.
2 Moxa the thorax and abdomen before the back and lumbar areas.

3 Use more moxa on the trunk than on the limbs and even less on the head and neck.

One almost invariably associates moxa with the application of heat, but similar effects can be achieved with the use of rubefacients and poultices, particularly those with a vesicatory action such as garlic paste or crushed castor oil seeds, whilst an interesting variation on the navel full of salt is to fill it with alum powder and then drip on cold water a drop at a time. This is used more especially for a heat syndrome with anuria and constipation.

A remaining consideration in the use of moxa is its use with a heated needle. This is achieved with either a piece of moxa punk wrapped round the handle, or a chunk of moxa roll about 1.5–2 cm long with a hole pierced through the centre and ignited from the bottom. The needle must be strong enough not to bend under the weight of the moxa and should therefore be about 28 gauge, placed deeply enough to hold firmly and long enough so that the burning moxa is at least 4 cm away from the skin surface. The Japanese actually produce ready-made small pieces of moxa roll about 13 mm long by about 13 mm in diameter with a hole already for placing on the handle of the needle. Unfortunately the hole is so large that the chunk slides down the handle and it is placed on the horizontal axis rather than the vertical one. This means that one has to produce another, smaller hole going through the other way! The Japanese also produce what are termed Fire Cups. These are little cups shaped rather like deep saucers which fit over the handle of the needle. They are then filled with moxa punk which is ignited. Unfortunately, unless the needle is absolutely vertical they invariably slide off and, being relatively heavy, they frequently bend the needle under their own weight with the same calamitous results. One therefore needs thick needles with relatively thin, smooth handles; these are not easily obtained and one cannot really recommend their use.

To shield the skin against any possible hot ash which might drop off onto the patient it is essential to use a guard, which is simply a piece of stout card with a hole pierced in the centre and dropped over the needle.

A technique which is almost the opposite to heating the handle of the needle is to place an ordinary filiform needle into the point and then heat the skin around the needle itself with a moxa roll. This naturally combines the sedative effect of the needle in situ with the warming effect (and therefore the capillary dilatory effect) of the moxa on the point. Its effect will thus be warming and sedatory.

Where there is Cold Bi, with stiff joints and crepitus, the particular effect of the so-called O/A technique, entailing alternating heat to the handle, must not be overlooked. The ordinary heated needle is extremely effective where there is a chronic degenerative condition or where there are fibrositic nodules, etc., when the local increase in circulatory (and other) changes will help to hasten the repair process.

There are two further uses for heated needles which need to be mentioned. One is in the case of spastic paralysis. In flaccid paralysis there is a deficiency of Yang, so ordinary moxa will suffice to bring this up to balance the Yin. In spastic paralysis, however, there is a normal Yang with an excess of Yin (see Newman Turner and Low, 1981). We must not drain the Yin so we have to reinforce the Yang to meet it, and this can best be done by inserting a needle into the appropriate point (especially GB34, Yanglingshuan), heating it with a spirit lamp until it is red hot, and withdrawing it while it is still glowing. The second further use is the Yuan-Li needle. This is used for benign swellings such as certain goitres and, particularly, ganglia and Baker's cysts, etc. The needle is thick, about 21 gauge, and 5.1 cm long. It is heated to a red/ white heat over a spirit lamp and then plunged swiftly into the centre of the swelling and immediately withdrawn. In some cases two or three treatments at roughly weekly intervals may be required.

8

The Plum-Blossom needle

Traditionally, the Plum-Blossom needle had five points, as against the Seven Star needle, which had seven. Nowadays most of the needles in use have seven points but all are known as Plum-Blossom needles!

There are two main types – the Hammer type and the Pipe type. The Hammer type is two-headed, with the seven-point star on one side of the head and either a conical point or a tight cluster of five small needles on the other, whilst the Pipe type consists of the seven-point star only. Because the same sterilization precautions should be observed as with ordinary needles, it is preferable for the whole needle (handle and head) to be made of metal, so that it can be placed in an autoclave. The only drawback to metal needles is that they are slightly heavy to handle. Needles of wood or wood and metal are freely available, but these tend to come apart when subjected to high temperatures, while plastic ones are far too flexible and in some cases do not respond well to the autoclave.

The indications for their use are particularly for children and those who are hypersensitive to pain, and they are particularly indicated in headaches, insomnia, dizziness and vertigo, gastrointestinal disorders, chronic disorders in women and some types of skin disease.

The handle should be held between the thumb and forefinger and stabilized against the palm with the other three fingers. If held too tightly it will cause muscular tension of the wrist with consequent loss of flexibility. If held too loosely the needle will tend to shake and rotate slightly and this can cause bleeding. The tip of the needle should be vertical to the skin and the tapping regular and accurate, coming from the wrist and lifted cleanly after each stroke. The frequency should be about 70–90 times a minute.

The intensity of stimulation is divided into three kinds:

1 Light – the wrist force is light and the force of impact is also small. Tap the local skin until it become erythematous.
2 Medium – using medium force tap the skin until it becomes red and purple but not bleeding.
3 Heavy – the wrist force and the force of impact are heavy. Tap the skin until it becomes very red and slight bleeding occurs.

Whether the tapping is light or heavy will depend upon the constitution of the patient, the nature of the disease and the regions to which it is applied. Generally, light tapping is used on the head and face, on the aged and weak, and on children. Medium tapping is used on general sites and generally, and heavy tapping is used on tender pressure points, the back and buttocks and on healthy adults of strong constitution, also on the solid hyperactive type of illness and in acute conditions.

One can of course use the Plum-Blossom needle to stimulate any acupuncture point as an alternative to the use of needles, but it is more specifically used for the stimulation of areas – either up or down the course of an aberrant meridian or to cover a specific area of the body, for example around the oral or mandibular regions in facial paralysis. Especially it is used to work down the sides of the spinal column, usually in three lines respectively 1, 2 and 3 cm away from the midline. Palpation of the areas on each side of the spine will often reveal increased tenderness, nodules or cord-like formations. These are indications of trouble in the organs pertaining to the related Back-Shu points and tapping should be performed on all three lines two to three times in these areas. This can be combined with tapping on the anterior aspect as follows:

- For diseases of the chest (including Ht and Lu disease) – along the intercostal space, along the sternum, costal angle and clavicular bone.
- For diseases of Liv, GB, Sp, St – from the costal angle down to the umbilicus horizontally and longitudinally, cross hammer 3–7 lines.
- For diseases of the intestines and genitourinary tract – from the umbilicus down to the upper edge of the pubis, horizontally and longitudinally, cross hammer 3–9 lines.
- For diseases of the genitalia – along the ilioinguinal canal, 1–2 lines.

There is a special technique, one that is particularly suitable for children, which involves the use of particular points on the vertebrae. It always begins with a stimulating action on the 'Universal Centre', GV7 (Zhongshu), between T10 and T11. Begin each treatment with stimulation of this point until the skin becomes red, then stop and continue by stimulation of the tips of the vertebrae as shown in Table 8.1 ('centre' refers to the very tip of the vertebra and 'sides' refers to the sides of the tip of the spinous process – see Fig. 8.1).

Similar in many respects to the Plum-Blossom needle in its usage is the 'rolling drum'. This, as its name implies, is a roller with a spiked surface which is rolled over the meridian or area where stimulation is

Table 8.1 Mai Hua technique

Region	Vertebrae	Remote areas (bilateral)
Head	C1 and C4, centre and sides	1st toe – lateral aspect (to 2nd)
Brain	C1 and C4, centre and sides	4th toe – lateral aspect
Cortex	C1 and C4, centre and sides	5th toe – lateral aspect
Hypophysis	C1 and C4, centre and sides	5th toe – lateral aspect
Face	C2 and C5 – sides only	None
Sense organs	Sides only	None
Scapula and upper limb	C5, C7 – sides only; D1 – centre and sides	None
Lungs, trachea and intercostals	C6, C7 – centre only; D1, D4 – centre and sides	Forearm along Lu line from wrist to elbow. Line must be red. Add scraping to pisiform bone at SI4 (Wangu)
Heart, diaphragm	D3, D6 – centre and sides	Forearm along Ht line, from elbow to wrist
St, Liv, GB, duodenum	D5, D9 – centre and sides	Along fibula (GB line) from head to malleolus. Add medial (internal) aspect 1st toe
SI (except duodenum), abdominal cavity, peritoneum	D8, D10 – centre and sides	None
Colon, anus	D9, D10, L3, L5, S2, S4 – centre and sides	None
Kidneys, urinary tract	D11, D12, L1, L2 – centre and sides	Sp9, also Heding point above patella
Bladder, female genitalia	L1–4 – centre and sides; whole of sacrum, especially the foramina	None

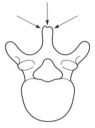

Figure 8.1

required. For mild stimulation the handle is held horizontally, whilst for a stronger effect the angle is increased to about 45°. The pressure can also be altered as required. The Japanese also produce a single needle mounted in a spring-loaded holder, which can be tapped over the area to produce superficial stimulation and erythema.

9

Cupping

One ancient method of treatment, widespread throughout the whole of Europe and Asia as well as China for many centuries, is the art of cupping. Like its contemporary treatment of bleeding by the use of leeches (now enjoying a resurgence in the Western world), it works by drawing blood to the area and thereby causing a movement in the blood and Qi, which will relieve stagnation and congestion.

To perform simple cupping a vessel containing a partial vacuum is placed over the designated area and the underlying superficial tissues are sucked up into the cup, the blood being brought to the surface in the process. Cups were originally made of horn or bamboo, but the preferred material these days is glass, which, being transparent, allows the operator to see what is happening to the skin. Pretty well any vessel of convenient size will do, such as a small jam jar, but a thickish rim is desirable as a thin one will tend to cut into the skin. Sets of ready-made cupping jars may now be purchased, consisting of small, medium and large cups; they are manufactured in both China and France and are naturally to be preferred.

There are several ways by which one can produce the desired partial vacuum, but the usual one is to take a piece of cotton wool, soak it in surgical spirit, wring it out and, holding it in a pair of forceps, set it alight and plunge it quickly into the cup, withdraw immediately and swiftly place the cup over the site. Another way, not used so much, is to soak a small piece of cotton wool in spirit, squeeze it out and place it on something small and non-combustible (usually a coin) over the spot. (As the coin can get hot, place it, in its turn, on a piece of thick card to protect the skin.) The cotton wool is then set alight and the cup placed over it – the burning cotton wool will exhaust the air.

Personally, I find it desirable to oil the skin first – olive oil is excellent – to give greater adherence. Warn the patient that a large bruise will result, but explain that this is not only normal but is actually desirable (being a sign that the treatment is working) and that it will disappear after three or four days. With subsequent treatment the bruising becomes less as the underlying congestion resolves.

The cup or cups are left on for 5–20 minutes depending upon the amount of discoloration appearing and the patient's somatotype. If left on for too long a blister may form. Small blisters may be disregarded, but larger ones should be punctured to remove the exudate and a dressing applied. Cups are removed by holding the cup with one hand and pressing down on the adjacent skin with the other, thus breaking the seal and loosening the cup.

As I have stated, cupping is used to get the Qi and blood moving. It is therefore used particularly for conditions of Qi and blood stagnation, poor circulation, asthmatic conditions, digestive problems and chronic low back pain due to Ki Xu. It is contraindicated over allergic skin conditions or where any skin lesions are present, in convulsions or cramps, in high fever or over the abdomen or low back during pregnancy. Care must be taken where the skin is thin, and the cups will not adhere over very hirsute areas or over bony prominences.

Where there is a large area of congestion and over thick muscles, as in low back spasms and similar states, a technique known as 'sliding' or 'migration' cupping is very useful. This means simply that instead of leaving the cup or cups in situ one slides the cup over the skin, the dermis being pulled up and loosened as the cup passes over and the circulation of the whole area being affected. To ensure continued adherence of the cup during this treatment Vaseline is often better than oil to lubricate the skin. (There is a Western variation on the standard cups obtainable whereby the vacuum is obtained by squeezing a rubber bulb attached to the bottom of the cup. These are often favourite for this particular technique as one can regulate the adherence so much more easily.)

Further variations include a combination of cupping with acupuncture, whereby a needle is inserted and a cup then placed over it whilst it is in place – this is particularly useful in rheumatic conditions. Another technique is that of 'wet-cupping' or 'scarification', whereby the skin is punctured (with a triangular needle or lancet) to induce bleeding and, instead of stopping the blood flow, the flow is encouraged by immediately placing a cup over the lesion to extract still more blood. This is useful in cases of neurodermatitis, pruritus, functional gastrointestinal diseases, etc., but always bear in mind the balance between blood and energy in the concerned meridian, and avoid bleeding where the blood content is weakest, i.e. Ki and Ht lines (see Chapter 6, 'Needle techniques').

10

Timing the treatment

Ideally, treatment should be given at a specific time on a specific date, as we will see shortly, according to what points are chosen, but this is invariably a policy of excellence which is very difficult to put into practice. Patients have to be seen when the practitioner can fit them in to a busy appointment schedule, and when they themselves can fit an appointment into their own schedule.

As I mention in my book *Acupuncture in Gynaecology and Obstetrics* (Low, 1990), in the part that deals with pulse diagnosis, the pulses should ideally be taken when the energies are as quiescent as possible, i.e. early in the morning before the Yang has had time to rise and stir things up. Woe betide the patient who breaks his fast with a cup of coffee and then dashes into the surgery because he is late for his appointment!

This means that when we take the pulses during our initial diagnosis we have to take several things into account. The Chinese Clock (see Fig. 10.1) is familiar to all acupuncturists.

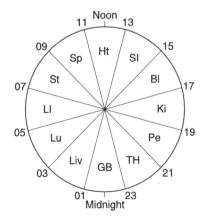

Figure 10.1

From this we could anticipate that the Spleen pulse would be dominant at 10.00 a.m., the Kidney at 6.00 p.m., etc., but equally, the Spleen would be full in the Late Summer and the Kidneys fullest in the Winter. The Liver pulse should be strong in the Spring, but a strong so-called 'hooky' Liver pulse is often associated with the presence of pain and this type of pulse can show up regardless of time or season.

Taking into account the fact that the Chinese season is six weeks ahead of ours, the typical pulses should be able to be described as follows:

- In Spring it is light and gliding.
- In Summer it is full and robust.
- In Autumn it is calm and rather superficial.
- In Winter it is hard and deep.

Forty-five days after the end of Winter the Yang energy rises softly to the distal wrist pulse, from the distal to the proximal pulse, then the Yin energy slowly descends. Forty-five days after the end of Summer the Yin energy slowly goes up to the distal pulse, then to the proximal pulse, then the Yang energy slowly descends.

According to some traditional statements one should not stimulate when the moon is full, nor in Spring or Summer. Similarly, one should not drain when the moon is empty or the room cold, nor in Autumn or Winter unless the moon is full and the room warm.

The energy potential increases in Spring, climaxes in Summer and decreases and remains in balance in Autumn, then reaches its minimum at the end of Winter. Therefore, as we prefer balances, the best season to treat general imbalances is in the Autumn (the 'season of needles'), i.e. September to December, when the energy is in equilibrium. General toning up gets its best results in the Chinese Spring, February to April, because at that time the natural movement of the energy is to increase. The best month for toning up is the end of February, because of the quick arrival of the Yang. December is the best for relaxing treatment, because of the quick arrival of the Yin.

Practitioners eventually develop an intuitive 'feel' for when the pulse is out of tune with its seasonal and hourly balance, but until such time they are advised to keep all the possible temporal divergences at the back of their mind and let the feel of the pulses impinge upon them. The pulse diagnosis is, of course, only a part of the attempt to arrive at an overall diagnostic picture, and both the Five Elements and the Eight Principles, plus the usual questions and examinations are simply pathways towards determining where the basic energic imbalance lies, and it is this which will decide our mode of treatment and the points selected.

But even when we have decided what we need to do there are still further temporal considerations. How a patient will respond to treatment will depend upon many factors. We are all aware of the traditional edicts which proscribe treatment during a thunderstorm, if the patient is drunk, if he is in any state of physical or mental unrest, etc. Anything like this can affect the circulation of energy in the physical/mental/emotional body, and just as disease can depend upon Internal or External 'devils', so the body's ability to react and respond to treatment will depend upon internal or external factors, and superimposed upon the reaction of the body as a whole is the variation in reaction of the meridians and the individual points.

We have already mentioned the Chinese Clock – the 24-hour cycle of energy – in connection with its effect upon the pulses. This, however, is a minor consideration compared with the actual ebb and flow of the energy in the meridians. The energy in any meridian is at its peak during its specific 2 hours out of the 24, and it is then that intervention in that particular meridian will have its maximum effect.

Employing natural movement is better than opposing it, therefore when we need to treat a weak patient it is better to stimulate between 5.00 a.m. and 3.00 p.m., when the energy normally increases, than later on when the energy is decreasing. Moreover, the best time for general toning is 11.00 a.m., when the Yin practically disappears, and the best time for general relaxation treatment is 5.00 p.m. when the Yang decreases.

On the other hand, the timetable in each meridian will help in organic treatments, because as the time flows, so a line is full or empty during the two precise hours – full for 2 hours and empty 12 hours later. For example, the Bladder is full at 3.00–5.00 p.m. and empty at 3.00–5.00 a.m.; the Stomach is full at 7.00–9.00 a.m. and empty at 7.00–9.00 p.m. Therefore, if we wish to stimulate or supply a meridian it is best to do it at the beginning of the flood time, i.e. Stomach at 7.00 a.m. and Bladder at 3.00 p.m. If we wish to drain or sedate at the end of the ebb tide this would be 9.00 p.m. for the Stomach and 5.00 a.m. for the Bladder.

Also to be taken into account is the so-called Midday/Midnight Law, which states that there is a relationship between organs which receive their maximum flow at opposed times; for example the Heart is maximum at 12.00 noon and the Gall Bladder at 12.00 midnight, the Stomach at 8.00 a.m. and the Pericardium at 8.00 p.m. The law states that an action taken on one organ will have an opposite action on the organ diametrically opposite it; i.e. tonifying the Heart will disperse the Gall Bladder. It is interesting to note that in every case a Yin organ is opposed by a Yang organ and vice versa, and the action is strongest if a Yin organ is stimulated in a

Yin time (midday to midnight) and a Yang organ in a Yang time (midnight to midday).

In practice it is found that only strong stimulation calls the law into effect – if an organ is given only moderate stimulation then that organ alone is affected. Also in practice, the energies do tend to equalize themselves, i.e. by tonifying the Spleen in the afternoon the Three Heaters would be sedated, but if the Three Heaters were in an already depleted state then tonification of the Spleen would tend to reinforce it and bring both Spleen and Three Heaters to a more balanced condition.

Generally, the Midday/Midnight Law is only applied when one wishes specifically to affect both the organ and its opposed organ in the appropriate ways. It will also be noted that in 50 per cent of the cases it conflicts with the use of the Horary points. Maximum effect would be achieved by using the Horary point of a Yang organ during the Yang period (i.e. Colon at 6.00 a.m., Stomach at 8.00 a.m.) or the Horary point of a Yin organ during the Yin period (i.e. Kidney at 6.00 p.m., Pericardium at 8.00 p.m.). Stimulating Sp3 at 10.00 a.m. would affect the Spleen strongly but would have a minimal effect on the Three Heaters, whereas stimulation of Sp2 at 6.00 p.m. would tonify the Spleen but also tend to disperse the Three Heaters.

Further concepts narrow the field still more, and it remains to consider the concept of the Celestial Stems. For a full understanding of this subject the student is referred to the author's book *The Celestial Stems* (Low, 1985b), but here we will simply state that just as the energy circulates in accordance with the kinetic Yang energy of the sun, so there is also a relationship with the lunar cycle upon which the old Chinese calendar was founded. Just as the moon affects the ebb and flow of the tides both in the external oceans and in the interior of our bodies, so it affects the energy in the different acupuncture points at specific times on specific days within the 60-day cycle. This means that individual points are 'open' or have their strongest effect at certain times, so that by utilizing this particular biorhythm one can achieve the most effective therapeutic result.

In the daily cycle the 'stems' are the days and the 'branches' are the 12 divisions of the 24 hours and the meridians pertaining thereto in their opening times (but please note that these are *not* the same as the 24-hour cycle we have already met). The Pericardium and Three Heaters do not appear in the column of opening times in Table 10.1 as they are functions rather than organs and obey their own rules. The energy slumbers between 11.00 p.m. and 3.00 a.m., when Yin is at its peak, and awakens in the Bladder with the opening of the eyes at 3.00 a.m. as in the circulation of the Tendino-Muscular meridians.

The overall calendric circulation is based on the 60-day cycle shown in Table 10.2.

Table 10.1 Opening days and times

Stems →			1	2	3	4	5	6	7	8	9	10
			Wo		F		E		M		Wa	
Opening Times →			Chia+	Yee–	Ping+	Ding–	Wu+	Ji–	Geng+	Shin–	Ren+	Gui–
			GB	Liv	SI	Ht	St	Sp	LI	Lu	Bl	Ki
2300–0100	Tzu+			SI2		SI4, LI3		GB38		St36		TH1
0100–0300	Chou–		Liv2		Liv3, Sp3		Ki7		Ht3		HC3	
0300–0500	Yin+	Bl		GB40, St43		Bl60		SI8		TH10	Bl67	
0500–0700	Mao–	Lu	HC7, Ki3, Ht7		Lu8		Liv8		HC5	Lu11		
0700–0900	Chen+	LI		LI5		GB34		TH6	LI1		GB43	
0900–1100	Si–	Sp	Sp5		Ki10		HC7	Sp1		Ki2		
1100–1300	Wu+	St		Bl40		TH3	St45		Bl66		Bl64, TH4, SI3	
1300–1500	Wei–	Ht	Lu5		Pe8	Ht9		Lu10		Lu9, Liv3	St41	(Sp5)
1500–1700	Shen+	SI		TH2	SI1	Sp2	LI2		LI4, GB41			
1700–1900	Yu–	Liv	HC9	Liv1				Sp3, Ki3		Ht4		(Lu5)
1900–2100	Shu+	GB	GB44		St44		St42, Bl65	Liv4	SI5		LI11	
2100–2300	Hai–	Ki		Ht8		Ht7, Lu9				Sp9		Ki1

Table 10.2 The Sixty-day Cycle

1	Chia-Tzu	21	Chia-Shen	41	Chia-Chen
2	Yee-Chu	22	Yee-Yu	42	Yee-Si
3	Ping-Yin	23	Ping-Shu	43	Ping-Wu
4	Ding-Mao	24	Ding-Hai	44	Ding-Wei
5	Wu-Chen	25	Wu-Tzu	45	Wu-shen
6	Ji-Si	26	Ji-Chou	46	Ji-Yu
7	Geng-Wu	27	Geng-Yin	47	Geng-Shu
8	Shin-Wei	28	Shin-Mao	48	Shin-Hai
9	Ren-Shen	29	Ren-Chen	49	Ren-Tzu
10	Gui-Yu	30	Gui-Si	50	Gui-Chou
11	Chia-Shu	31	Chia-Wu	51	Chia-Yin
12	Yee-Hai	32	Yee-Wei	52	Yee-Mao
13	Ping-Tzu	33	Ping-Shen	53	Ping-Chen
14	Ding-Chou	34	Ding-Yu	54	Ding-Si
15	Wu-Yin	35	Wu-Shu	55	Wu-Wu
16	Ji-Mao	36	Ji-Hai	56	Ji-Wei
17	Geng-Chen	37	Geng-Tzu	57	Geng-Shen
18	Shin-Si	38	Shin-Chou	58	Shin-Yu
19	Ren-Wu	39	Ren-Yin	59	Ren-Shu
20	Gui-Wei	40	Gui-Mao	60	Gui-Hai

To find out which of the actual Chinese days we are concerned with, the following calculation has to be performed:

1 Each year is given a 'root number' for the Stem and Branch of that year. This number increases by a factor of 5 for each year, except for the year following a Leap Year when 6 is added. (When the cycle of 60 years is completed, it recommences.) For example, the root numbers for the years 1991 to 2001 are given in Table 10.3.

2 Each month is also given a root number, as shown in Table 10.4.

Table 10.3

Year	1991	1992	1993	1994	1995	1996	1997	1998	1999	2000	2001
Root number	7	12	18	23	28	33	39	44	49	54	60
		↑				↑				↑	
		Leap year				Leap year				Leap year	

Table 10.4

Month	1	2	3	4	5	6	7	8	9	10	11	12
Normal year	0	31	59	30	0	31	1	32	3	33	4	34
Leap year	0	31	0	31	1	32	2	33	4	34	5	35

The reader will see that this is obtained simply by adding on the days of the preceding month of the year and deducting 60 whenever the 60-day cycle is completed.

The formula is simply to add the root number of the year to the root number of the month, plus the number of the day of the month as shown in the following examples.

14 March 1991

1991		March		14				
7	+	59	+	14	=	80	=	20 on 60-day cycle; and no. 20 on our chart is Gui-Wei

27 November 1996 (a leap year)

1996		November		27						
33	+	11	+	27	=	71 (less 60)	=	11	=	Chia-Shu

The duplex Stem-Branch will actually give us the specific year in the 60-year cycle; the name of the Stem alone will tell us which day it is in the 10-day cycle.

11

Finding the point

The fundamental requirements of an acupuncture practice are firstly a diagnosis and secondly the decision as to what point to use. But no matter how precise one is in arriving at the correct formula, it is all to no avail if the position of the point is not accurate enough to produce the required reaction on the part of the body/mind complex.

One of the most frequent questions put by patients is 'How big is the point and how accurate does the practitioner have to be?' The answer, as with so many acupuncture questions, is not quite so precise as one would wish: 'It all depends . . .' It depends upon the physical build of the patient, on the state of his/her basic energy, and on the season of the year. This latter is an important consideration because the energy goes deep in the Winter, like the seed buried in the soil to await the arrival of the Spring, and everything becomes condensed. One can picture it as in Fig. 11.1, so that in Winter one has not only to go deeper with the needle, but one has to be far more precise with the needling.

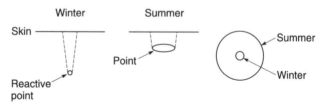

Figure 11.1

In Summer the energy has come more to the surface and the reactive energy has tended to spread out more, so that one's needling should be more superficial and, although one should endeavour to be as precise as possible, one can produce a reaction from a bigger area around the actual points. (One has to remember that although one refers to the point as if it is a material entity, this is only a working concept, as it is in reality only a nexus of energy – albeit one which can be readily detected by electrical means.)

Further to this there are considerations of the Five Elements to be taken into account (Fig. 11.2).

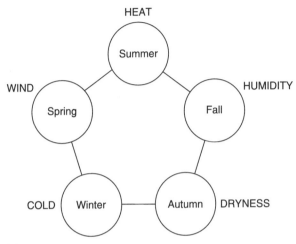

Figure 11.2

The seasons also correlate with the tissues:

Spring   –   Epidermis
Summer   –   Flesh
Autumn   –   Muscle
Winter   –   Bone

In Spring the Wind, or Fong, is the most prevalent Perverse Energy, but also the energy of the Liver begins to predominate; its energy is very full, consequently the perverse Fong cannot penetrate very deeply. It will produce superficial symptoms such as sneezing, blocked or running nose, headache and possibly coughs, and if it goes deeper can affect the Dai Yang with fever, fear of cold, perspiration, headache and signs of affection of the Small Intestine and Bladder meridians such as trapezial fibrosis and muscular problems on their pathway, etc.

In Spring the Yin energy of the body, like that of the earth, is rising again, and it will therefore be found in the superficial tissues and the Tendino-Muscular (T/M) meridians. (Students will often point out that the T/M meridians contain Wei energy, so how could there be Yin energy in them? Yin is the potential, Wei energy is the defensive aspect, the primary physiological response, but without Yin there could be no Wei, so that in the T/Ms the Yin has now assumed its kinetic aspect and is *functioning* as Wei.)

The Perverse Energy attacking the superficial regions pursues the Wei energy as far as the Tsing (Jing Well) point. It cannot invade further because of the growing strength of the Jung energy in the main meridian. Treatment could therefore consist of the use of the T/M technique – puncture painful points in the area, stimulate the Tsing point, and support the principal meridian concerned via its tonification point.

In Summer the energy of the Heart is strong, though not so strong as the Yong energy of the body. This latter, originally superficial in the Spring, goes deeper into the tissues (Flesh) and penetrates the meridians as far as the Yong (Ying) points. As it is strong it is also found in the Luo vessels, and from these it can enter into the principal meridian. Perverse Energy enters into the body by the same route – T/Ms and Luos – up to the Yong point. It must not be allowed to get beyond this because at the Yu (Shu) point it would be absorbed for carriage elsewhere (see Chapter 2, on the 'Welling' Theory). We must therefore drain the Yu points to prevent this happening, whilst we would also treat the Luo point of the same meridian.

In Autumn the Yang energy begins to decline and become more Yin. The Perverse Energy of Humidity is the most prevalent, and this is in itself of a Yin nature, but there is still enough Yang energy present to prevent it penetrating into the deeper levels of the organs. According to Chamfrault, to whom much of this work can be attributed, at this point the Yang energy penetrates into the main meridian via the normal channels (T/Ms and Luos) up to the Ching (Jing River) point where:

- in a Yin meridian the Yang energy weakens and is dispersed into nearby bone, muscle, etc.;
- in a Yang meridian the Yang energy goes on to the Ho (He) point, where it collects before either dispersing into the region or going deep to the viscera.

Perverse Energy follows the same course and we therefore drain the Ching point. The Yu point is the point of entry of Perverse Energy and also of Wei energy, therefore by combining the Ching with the Yu points we call on the defensive energy and activate Wei towards the affected region.

Therefore, in all affections of the 'Yin in the Yang' (bones, muscles, marrow, etc.) it pays to consider the use of the Ching and the Yu points. However, the Su Wen (the first part of the *Nei Ching*) advises in Chapter 73 the Ching point plus either the Yu point of a Yin meridian or the Ho point of a Yang meridian.

In Winter the body's Yang becomes very feeble (quiescent) whilst the Yin becomes correspondingly strong. Traditionally, needles were not used much during this season because, as the Yin energy predominates and 'Yin engenders the Yang', puncturing the Yin harms the Yang. Also, the prevailing Perverse Energies are usually of a Cold nature, and the use of moxibustion would be naturally called for.

The Su Wen says: 'In Winter the Yang is weak and deep, and the Kidneys close their gates. The Kidneys are the gates (barriers) of the Stomach. With poor functioning the water accumulates and overflows'. Therefore an attack by Cold/Wind may cause oedema. In this case, Yin energy must be drawn to the lower part of the body and made to enter into the meridian by puncturing the Tsing point, *but* there is already an excess of Yin in the lower part of the body, so the Yang, already weak, would become even weaker. We must therefore support the Yang by puncturing the Yong points to draw the defensive Yang which participates in the defence of the organism against Perverse Energy. In Winter, therefore, we use the Tsing and Yong points, and these points are always useful to remember in cases of oedema due to Wind/Cold.

Returning to the question of the exact position of the points, the Chinese literature invariably states that the point lies in a specific place and at a specific depth. To determine the place anatomically they long ago devised the concept of the Chinese (or acupuncture) inch, or cun. This was an ingenious method of taking into account the various sizes and builds of patients and was based upon the patient's

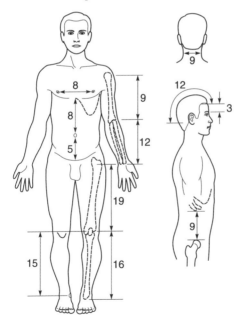

Figure 11.3

own anatomy. It consisted of selecting two anatomical landmarks and dividing the distance between them into a certain number of units, so it is applicable to any patient – short or tall, young or old, slim or obese, male or female. The system in common use can be seen with the aid of Fig. 11.3.

On the skull we assign a measurement of 12 cun to the distance along the midline from the hairline over the forehead to the inion at the back of the head. If the front hairline is hard to distinguish, measure from the glabella, the midpoint between the eyebrows, and add 3 cun, making 15 in all.

A second common method is to base the cun upon the length of the middle phalanx of the patient's middle finger, by placing the tip of the patient's middle finger against the tip of their thumb to form a ring, and then measuring the distance between the wrinkles at the first and second joints of the finger, as shown in Fig. 11.4.

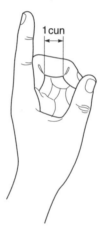

Figure 11.4

One thing I have found to be extremely annoying in many of the Chinese books, is where they describe one point as being so many cun distal or proximal to some other point, which means that if you get the first point wrong, then the other is automatically also in the wrong place.

Personally, I prefer to stick purely to anatomical landmarks, bony ridges, etc. and to look for easily divisible measurements which can be split into equal portions between the practitioner's outstretched fingers. As an example, the distance between the sterno-xiphoid junction and the umbilicus (CV8) is 8 cun. Splitting this into half would locate CV12 (at 4 cun above CV8) and also Ki19 and Sp21 on the same level. Splitting the upper half, between CV12 and CV16, gives us CV14 and the levels of Ki21, St19 and (roughly) Liv14. Splitting the lower half between CV12 and CV8 gives us CV10, Ki17 and St23, and each of these halves can be further split for CV9 and CV11 and the appropriate points on their level.

The distance between the umbilicus (CV8) and the pubic symphysis is 5 cun, which is difficult to split precisely, and one therefore has to estimate halfway as $2\frac{1}{2}$ cun, halfway down to the symphysis is $1\frac{1}{4}$ cun, and $\frac{4}{5}$ of this is 1 cun up, which is CV3. One can then easily split the remaining 4 cun for the other CV points and the points on their level.

On the arm, the lower arm at 12 cun is ideal as it is so easy to split half and then quarters – LI6, TH6, TH7 and Pe5 distally, LI8 at 4 cun proximally and estimate Lu6 at 5 cun below the cubital fossa.

For the upper arm, with 9 cun from the level of the top of the axillary crease to the tip of the epicondyle, we easily estimate thirds, to get Lu3 at 3 cun 'down', Ht2 at 3 cun 'up' and LI13 laterally.

Measurements for the points on the lower leg are preferably taken on the lateral aspect, where from the femoro-tibial junction it is 16 cun to the tip of the lateral malleolus, whereas on the medial aspect to the tip of the medial malleolus it is 15 cun. Sixteen cun can be halved to 8, giving us St40, St38, Bl57 and Liv6. Halfway between this and the malleolus, i.e. 4 cun 'up', is GB38 and, sliding over to the medial side of the tibia, Sp6. Fixing Sp6 with one's index finger, reach out and down to one-third the distance to the medial malleolus with the middle finger and one is on Ki7 and the level of Ki8. Still on the medial aspect, it is easy to estimate one-third 'down' – fix the upper and lower limits with your little fingers and mark the junction of the upper and lower thirds with the index fingers to find Sp8 and Liv5. (As noted above, Liv6 is more accurately found from the level of St40.) Superior to St40 we halve and halve again for St37. This process can be extended to the whole of the body, with the exception of those points that lie in definite hollows such as LI4, LI11, LI15, TH14, SI10, Lu2 and GB34 and similar. GB30 is one-third of the way between the tip of the great trochanter and the sacro-coccygeal junction. (An interesting note here is that there is an internal pathway between GB30 and St30, and St30 is the beginning of a secondary vessel of Chong Mai – and the Su Wen states 'In all cases of paralysis or other troubles of the legs, think of St30'!)

A further point of interest is that pain radiating down the Bladder line is on the distribution of the first sacral nerve, which emerges at the lumbo-sacral junction and therefore calls for concentration on the special point Shiqizhui at its L5/S junction, and the use of such of the affected points Bl36, 37, 39, 40, 57, 58 and 60 and GB41 and 43 as may be called for.

For sciatica with a lateral leg distribution we are concerned with the fifth lumbar nerve which emerges in the region of L4/5 (thus GV3) and affects Bl25, GB30, 31, 34, 36, 37, 39 and St 41, Liv3 and Liv2.

There remains to mention the use of measurement which equates the cun with the width of the operator's fingers. This is extremely unreliable as is the use of the electrical point detector – this latter because any slight presence of moisture on the skin will give a false reading. Moreover, swabbing the skin with ether to dry it will give a false reading, as will passing over the point more than once – the previous pressure will affect the result.

Having detected where the point is, there still remains the *exact* determination, and this will depend upon the operator's sensitivity. The majority of points lie in little hollows either between the bones or in between the muscle planes, and the finger rolls into them, but we mentioned earlier that there is a change in electrical resistance over the points. This is detectable by the finger – a slight 'tackiness' is the only way to describe it, almost a 'buzzing', as the tip (or actually the pulp) of the finger is passed *very lightly* over the point. The intensity can tell one the degree of activity within the point, which with practice can even be detected without actually touching the area – but this brings us into the realms of Qi Kung, which is a separate study.

12

Formulating a treatment

We have dealt at some length with the many considerations involved in point selection. Many and detailed as these may appear, to a competent acupuncturist they should all be present in the back of the mind, so that the appropriate ones are subconsciously brought to bear while assessing the patient.

The basic diagnosis will decide whether we are going to put the emphasis on local or systemic treatment – if the patient comes in complaining of pain in the cervical area radiating down the arm coming on after a shunt in his or her car, I am going to concentrate on the treatment of a possible whiplash injury, i.e. purely locally with the use of local and distant points. I would not anticipate any variation on the pulse or tongue (unless the patient is suffering from secondary shock or a vasomotor dysfunction), neither would I anticipate any Zang/Fu syndromes. Don't start talking about stagnation of blood or Qi – of course there is, but stimulation of CV4 or 6 won't do a thing. Consider rather whether needles or moxa might possibly be less effective than massage or neuromuscular techniques, or even interferential therapy, and if there is a lesion present, are you capable of diagnosing it and, once diagnosed, of correcting it?

However, if the patient comes in with an obviously systemic condition, then the pulse and tongue are primary sources of information as we think first of the overall pulse picture, i.e. the Eight-Principle one, and then break it down to palpation of the individual pulses to see if any specific imbalances can be determined. If there are, we then have to decide whether to pursue a Five-Element pathway and correct the imbalance between the organs as in Chapter 2, or use the more general Eight-Principle one of a treatment for the prevailing syndrome. The whole general picture will point the practitioner to the major element concerned, but he or she then has to decide whether to treat by putting the emphasis on the element or the symptom pattern.

In other words, if the patient presents with a lung condition, does one treat the lung organ and/or the meridian, or the symptoms as presented by a Traditional Chinese Medicine (TCM) diagnosis?

Basically, treatment may be regarded as being of three types:

1 Direct
2 Semi-direct
3 Indirect

Direct treatment consists of using points actually on the concerned principal meridian alone, to affect purely that meridian and its concerned organ. Semi-direct means that one utilizes the Back Shu and Front Mu points to affect the organ and hence the meridian. (Note: traditionally this is semi-direct, but I personally feel that the Back Shu points have a more direct effect upon the organ than do any other points.) Indirect infers that we use 'command points' on other meridians for their effect upon the meridian being treated, for example use of points on the Colon meridian to affect its coupled Lung meridian (see also the use of the Antique Points in Chapter 3).

This latter basically relates to the symptom-pattern approach of TCM, where after careful case-taking one arrives at a diagnosis of a specific Zang/Fu syndrome and devises a particular formula to correct that syndrome pathology. At this point one must note that a TCM diagnosis is based upon completely different premises from those prevailing in Western medicine, and the treatment must be based upon those different premises. It is that particular syndrome that we are trying to correct, not a diagnosis based upon laboratory reports, and adherence to the TCM principles is the only way to achieve success if that is the route we have chosen.

However, it must be stressed that, as I stated at the very beginning, in my opinion (and experience) TCM is an elementary approach to a lot of the problems with which we are confronted, and is not always the most effective. In purely systemic conditions an approach via the element is frequently more fundamental and more effective. To stand back and attempt to get a mental picture of what is happening to the actual energy and its circulation in the patient's body is to practise acupuncture as it should be practised, and is the way to produce those occasional truly amazing results which make the practitioner's lot so satisfying and rewarding.

A simple illustration of this would be one in which the patient presents with the very typical picture – somewhat overweight, heavy and waterlogged in the lower part of the body, panting, wheezing and over-encumbered in the upper part. This is the classical picture of too much energy (albeit a blocked Yang trying to get an overworked heart and lungs to function properly) up above, and not enough (albeit an excess Yin condition – note Yin condition, not Yin energy) down below. We have to relieve the heart and lungs, but they are weakened already, so we cannot just go draining willy-nilly, yet if we moxa to strengthen them we could increase the false fire and aggravate the symptoms. We have to get the energy moving in the lower part and encourage the kidneys to get rid of the excess fluid. Obviously there is a basic Kidney weakness, and a typical approach would be to moxa Bl23 (Shenshu), Ki3 (Taixi), Ki7 (Fuliu), etc. But surely one of the essential considerations is to obey the basic rule of getting the energy to flow from an excess to a deficiency. Ki7 would do that (stimulate, not moxa, because we are 'pulling' the energy to a degree) by transferring from Lu to Ki on the Sheng cycle. But a more direct way would be to 'loosen the belt' by the use of Dai Mai, the girdle vessel, and pull the energy down by stimulating St39 (Xiajuxu). Note that the lower Ho points have a further function than that of being the Ho points for SI and LI – St37 (Shangjuxu) is for 'too much energy in the upper part of the body', St39 (Xiajuxu) is for 'not enough energy in the lower part of the body'. Only after we have tried this fundamental approach should we embark on other more local treatments of TCM.

Students are often confused by being taught that the Yang energy rises whilst the Yin descends. This is the opposite to their correct flow – Yang flows downwards from the energies of Heaven, Yin flows upwards from the Earthly nourishment, and Man is the resultant balance in between.

The energic movements in the body are governed from the centre (in Japanese acupuncture the Hara), because it is from here that the energies of Blood and Air are distributed to the periphery. The points commanding the distribution (Fig. 12.1) are:

- CV12 (Zhongwan) to distribute the energy.
- LI10 (Shousanli) for the upper part of the body and upper limbs.
- St36 (Zusanli) for the lower part of the body and lower limbs.

(Note how these last two points are called San Li, 'three paths' – of energy, blood and air.)

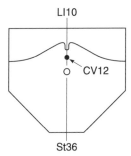

Figure 12.1

The pelvis

The pelvis is the most Yin zone of the body. Where energy is concerned we have to consider its intensity and its movements.

Intensity

We have seen that the Yang energy descends, so its intensity is most characteristic in the Tai Yang and the thorax, it is of medium intensity in the Shao Yang and the supra-umbilical region, and least characteristic in the Yang Ming to end in the pelvic region. The point commanding the end of Yang in the pelvic basin is St29 (Guilai).

Yin energy, which ascends, is Tai Yin in the pelvis, Shao Yin in the supra-umbilical region and Jueh Yin where it ends in the thoracic region (Fig. 12.2).

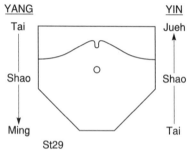

Figure 12.2

Movement

The references used here are Shao, the youngest, Tai, the greatest, and Jueh or Ming, the ending or finishing, and the command points for the areas are for the descending Yang St29 (Guilai), and for the ascending Yin Ki13 (Qixue) (Fig. 12.3).

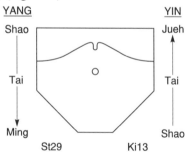

Figure 12.3

Barriers

The pelvic region is in close relationship with the inferior members (the legs). A pathology at the barrier at the level of the hip can cause pathological repercussion in the pelvis, especially in the case of a movement of Yin or Yang energy into the lower limbs. If the hip joint is blocked with Yang, the Yang energy of the pelvic basin cannot flow into the lower limbs and will be in excess in the pelvis, whilst a blockage of Yin energy will cause an excess of Yin in the basin.

The command point to move the Yang is Bl29 (Zhanglushu) and to move the Yin is Sp12 (Chongmen) (Fig. 12.4).

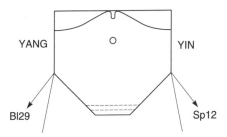

Figure 12.4

At the level of the whole body

To be considered in those cases where pelvic troubles are not isolated but are associated with trouble in the trunk generally.

Intensity (Fig. 12.5)
> Yang energy is Tai at the level of the upper limbs
> Yang energy is Shao at the level of the trunk
> Yang energy is Ming at the level of the lower limbs
> (Inverse for the Yin energy)

Movement (Fig. 12.6)
> Yang energy is Shao at the level of the upper limbs
> Yang energy is Tai at the level of the trunk
> Yang energy is Ming at the level of the lower limbs

When the energy is moved we have an interchange between up and down, and between the interior and the exterior.

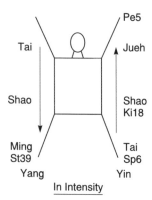

Figure 12.5

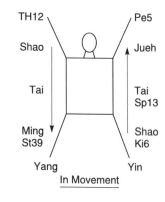

Figure 12.6

Up and down:

Yang must go down (Shao Yang – TH12, augment with St39).
Yin must go up (when Yin plus below, Shao Yin – Ki6 and Pe5).

When Dai Mai 'tight' it blocks the energy (Yang and Yin) giving stagnation of Yin below and stagnation of Yang above. We must therefore open Dai Mai using GB26, GB41 and TH5.

Internal and external:

The internal is Chong Mai and Blood energy (St). When blood and energy are blocked inside there is nothing in the extremities. When energy is blocked in the limbs, then there is a deficiency in the trunk. We therefore make use of the treatment mentioned earlier:

   CV12 to distribute the energy;
   LI10 to attract it to the arms;
   St36 to attract it to the legs.

Barrier points are to be used when energy is blocked in the articulations. They always react via the rules of:
Before the block – fullness; after the block – emptiness.
   Troubles with the exit of energy give empty Yang symptoms (e.g. in hands we could get cold fingers), generally better by pressure and heat and more likely right-sided; or empty Yin symptoms, which are better by pressure and cold and tending to the left side. Troubles with the entry give Yin or Yang fullness. Use the Yin or Yang barrier points accordingly (Fig. 12.7).

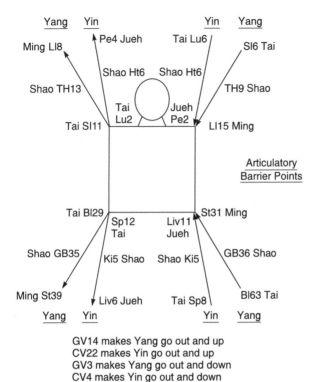

GV14 makes Yang go out and up
CV22 makes Yin go out and up
GV3 makes Yang go out and down
CV4 makes Yin go out and down

Figure 12.7

Superficial and deep

Figure 12.8 recapitulates energy movement within the six Chiaos.

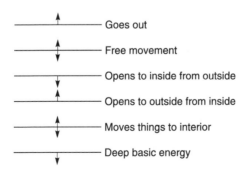

Figure 12.8

Movement from out to in:

- To bring Yang in – St25.
- To bring Yin in – CV3.
- To start Yang in general – GB25.
- To bring Yin out – GB24, strengthened with GB23.
- To bring Yang out – CV17, brings up to Tai Yang level.

The Liv is the main meridian in the leg in which Jueh Yin energy circulates and in which all Jueh Yin phenomena are found.

- To command whole energy in intensity Liv10 (distributes Yin/Yang energy).
- Emergence point – Liv11.
- Emerging points dealing with spacial conditions – Liv7, Liv9, Liv13.
- Emerging points dealing with time conditions – Liv14 (Liv10 when empty Yin in the centre).
- Liv11 – Small Yin coming in, facilitates entry of Yin of leg into the trunk.
- Liv12 – Luo point of genital organs.

The pelvis is the most Yin part of the body, so should have free movement of Yin. When there is blockage we get constipation, dysmenorrhoea, lumbago, polyuria and cold – use Liv9. Liv13 is the barrier point for the trunk and distributes Yin from the centre to the periphery (Yin blockage in trunk). It always has a relationship with the Spleen.

When troubles with Time are concerned (Shao-Tai-Jueh), Jueh is the end, so use Liv14, which should be considered for all troubles concerning the end of movement.

Many of the foregoing concepts owe their promulgation to doctors teaching in France – writers and lecturers such as Doctors Andrès, Kespi, Rocher, Roustan, Minh and Savigny – but the original theories of energetic movements are founded upon Vietnamese teachings, which are themselves based on the purest of traditional Chinese acupuncture.

Also to be considered when thinking in terms of the global movement of energy are the points with a special action mentioned in Chapter 4, particularly the Windows of the Sky and the Points of the Four Seas. It is this overall 'global' view which enables us to appreciate that most valid of all Chinese statements: 'The Master will never use two needles where one will do, but that one needle must be expertly placed in both place and time'; and it is this method of practice which, as we have said, can prove so satisfying for the practitioner.

Once the decision has been made as to what needs to be done, it is then simple to decide which method of treatment we are going to adopt from the various means at our disposal – global, Five Elements (Phases), Eight Principles, etc., or even purely local. If going by the TCM pathway, almost every book emanating from China contains lists of the functions of the points, as in the notes on 'Pathogenic relationships' in Chapter 4, and one uses one's knowledge of these to affect any disturbance of the Zang/Fu and their syndromes. A disturbance affecting the meridians leads us to consider which points can have the strongest effect, and here the concept of the Welling Theory is of great value. As an example, the simple fact that the Perverse Energy escapes at the Ching point into the neighbouring joints and tissues tells us that these points can be of immense use when treating any conditions of these structures. We should also consider the reunion points.

Particularly when dealing with musculo-skeletal problems we will find that our knowledge of Western medicine, in particular the dermatomal and nerve distribution, is of value. Taking a simple case of sciatica, from an acupuncture viewpoint the most common radiation would be down either the lateral aspect of the leg or down the posterior, i.e. either the GB or Bl (UB) lines. However, our anatomical knowledge will tell us that the lateral distribution is of the fifth lumbar nerve, originating mainly from L4/5 or GV3 (Yaoyangguan), whilst the posterior distribution comes mainly from the first sacral nerve at L5/S1 (Shiqizhui).

A further study of the dermatomes will show us that the fifth lumbar nerve will comprehend the acupuncture points of GV3, Bl25 (Dachangshu), GB30 (Huantiao), GB31 (Fengshi), GB34 (Yanglingquan), GB36 (Waiqiu), GB37 (Guangming), GB39 (Xuanzhong), GB40 (Qiuxu), St41 (Jiexi), Liv3 (Taichong) and the two medial Bafeng points, whilst the first sacral nerve, from Shiquizhui, will embrace Bl26 (Guanyuanshu), Huanzhong midway between GB30 and GV2 (Yaoshu), but then usually passes lateral to the Bladder meridian. The actual Bladder points that can be used could comprise Bl36 (Chengfu), Bl37 (Yinmen), Bl39 (Weiyang), Bl40 (Weizhong), Bl57 (Chengshan), Bl58 (Feiyang), Bl60 (Kunlun), with GB41 (Linqi) and the two lateral Bafeng points. But to utilize the more lateral path of the dermatome three non-meridial points have been discovered on the posterior thigh – Jianbu, 2 cun lateral to Bl36 (Chengfu), Jianzhong 2 cun lateral to Bl37 (Yinmen), and Jianxia, 2 cun below Jianzhong. A useful point to consider in sciatica is GB39 (Xuanzhong) as it is the group Luo point affecting all the Yang meridians of the leg, just as Sp6 (Sanyinjiao) affects all the three Yin.

Earlier on I stated that the Master would never use two needles where one would do, yet in the example above I proceed to use any or all of 14 points for a simple sciatica. Really, of course, one would select from the most appropriate of the points at the time of treatment, but basically it serves to illustrate the different mode of thought employed when treating a systemic imbalance – find the root cause and treat that, possibly 'swinging' the imbalance over with the one needle 'expertly applied' – and when treating a mechanical dysfunction, where we may possibly need the accumulative effect of 'points in line' to induce strong endorphin anti-inflammatory action.

All of which boils down to the simple fact that the essence of point selection is feeling. Learn every possible approach, the function of every point, then empty them out of your mind and tune in to the patient. It is similar to when one is palpating an abdomen – never tell yourself 'I am looking for an ovarian cyst'. Empty your mind, and then ask yourself 'What does this abdomen tell me?'

References and further reading

Academies of Chinese Medicine (1987) *Chinese Acupuncture and Moxibustion.* Beijing: Foreign Languages Press.

Academies of Chinese Medicine (1989) *Essentials of Contemporary Chinese Acupuncturists' Clinical Experiences.* Beijing: Foreign Languages Press.

Baldry, P. E. (1989) *Acupuncture Trigger Points and Musculoskeletal Pain.* Edinburgh: Churchill Livingstone.

Bensoussan, A. (1991) *The Vital Meridian.* Edinburgh: Churchill Livingstone.

Chamfrault, A. (1964) *Traité de Médecine Chinoise.* Angoulême: Editions Coquemard.

Chamfrault, A. and Van Nghi, N. (1975) *L'Energetiques Humaine en Médecine Chinoise.* Angoulême: Imprimerie de la Charante.

Kaptchuk, T. (1983) *The Web that has no Weaver.* New York: Congdon and Weed.

Lavier, J. Personal communications.

Lee, J. F. and Cheung, C. S. (1978) *Current Acupuncture Theory.* Hong Kong: Medical Interflow.

Low, R. (1983) *The Secondary Vessels of Acupuncture.* Wellingborough: Thorsons.

Low, R. (1985a) *Acupuncture Atlas and Reference Book.* Wellingborough: Thorsons.

Low, R. (1985b) *The Celestial Stems.* Wellingborough: Thorsons.

Low, R. (1987) *The Acupuncture Treatment of Musculo-Skeletal Conditions.* Wellingborough: Thorsons.

Low, R. (1988) *The Non-Meridial Points of Acupuncture.* Wellingborough: Thorsons.

Low, R. (1990) *Acupuncture in Gynaecology and Obstetrics.* London: Thorsons.

Lu Gwei-Djen and Needham, J. (1980) *Celestial Lancets.* Cambridge: Cambridge University Press.

Matsumoto, K. and Birch, S. (1983) *Five Elements and Ten Stems.* Brookline, MA: Paradigm Publications.

Needham, J. (1962) *Science and Civilisation in China,* Vols 2 and 3. Cambridge: Cambridge University Press.

Nei Ching (Su Wen, Ling Shu, Nan Ching) (1978) [complete translation by Henry Lu]. Vancouver: Academy of Oriental Heritage.

Newman Turner, R. and Low, R. (1981) *Principles and Practice of Moxibustion.* Wellingborough: Thorsons.

O'Connor, J. and Bensky, D. (1981) *Acupuncture, a Comprehensive Text.* Chicago, IL: Eastland Press.

Porkert, M. (1974) *Theoretical Foundations of Chinese Medicine.* Cambridge, MA: MIT Press.

Porkert, M. (1983) *Essentials of Chinese Diagnosis.* Zurich: Acta Medicinae Sinensis.

Ross, J. (1987) *Zang/Fu.* Edinburgh: Churchill Livingstone.

Seem, M. (1987) *Acupuncture Energetics.* Wellingborough: Thorsons.

Seem, M. (1993) *A New American Acupuncture.* Boulder, CT: Blue Poppy Press.

Shudo Denmei (1990) *Introduction to Meridian Therapy.* Seattle: Eastland Press.

Yamashita, M. (1971) *Introductory Text of Acupuncture for Meridian Therapy.* Tokyo.

Index